# PRINCIPLES AND TECHNIQUES IN ONCOPLASTIC BREAST CANCER SURGERY

# PRINCIPLES AND TECHNIQUES IN ONCOPLASTIC BREAST CANCER SURGERY

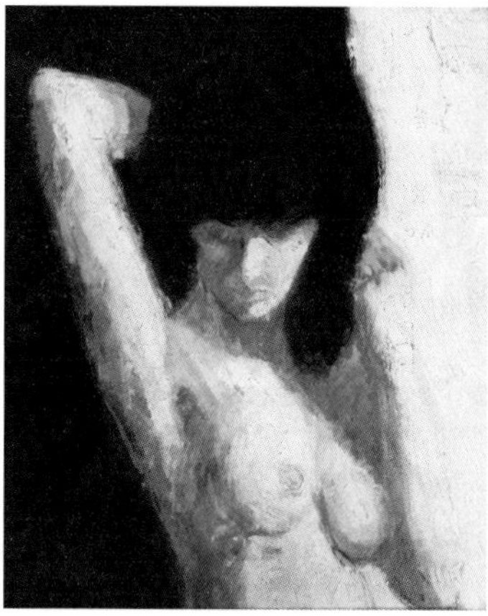

Editor

**Mahmoud Bahij El-Tamer**, MD, FACS

Memorial Sloan-Kettering Cancer Center & Cornell University, USA

World Scientific

NEW JERSEY • LONDON • SINGAPORE • BEIJING • SHANGHAI • HONG KONG • TAIPEI • CHENNAI

*Published by*

World Scientific Publishing Co. Pte. Ltd.
5 Toh Tuck Link, Singapore 596224
*USA office:* 27 Warren Street, Suite 401-402, Hackensack, NJ 07601
*UK office:* 57 Shelton Street, Covent Garden, London WC2H 9HE

**British Library Cataloguing-in-Publication Data**
A catalogue record for this book is available from the British Library.

**PRINCIPLES AND TECHNIQUES IN ONCOPLASTIC BREAST CANCER SURGERY**



ISBN 978-981-4327-76-3

Typeset by Stallion Press
Email: enquiries@stallionpress.com

Printed in Singapore by Mainland Press Pte Ltd.

To Hania, Bahij, Sarah, my parents, and my siblings, for all your unconditional support.

# CONTENTS

# LIST OF CONTRIBUTORS

Jeffrey Ascherman, MD
Professor of Clinical Surgery
Division of Plastic Surgery
New York-Presbyterian Hospital/Columbia
New York, NY, USA.

Susan K. Boolbol, MD
Chief, Division of Breast Surgery
Beth Israel Medical Center
New York, NY 10003, USA.

Adriana D. Corben, MD
Director, Breast Pathology Fellowship Program
Department of Pathology
Memorial Sloan-Kettering Cancer Center
New York, NY 10065, USA.

Mahmoud Bahij El-Tamer, MD, FACS
Breast Service, Department of Surgery
Memorial Sloan-Kettering Cancer Center
Professor of Clinical Surgery
Weill Medical College at Cornell University
New York, NY 10065, USA.

Sheldon Feldman, MD
Chief, Division of Breast Surgical Oncology
Columbia University Medical Center
New York City, NY 10032, USA.

Tara L. Huston, MD
Assistant Professor of Surgery
Division of Plastic and Reconstructive Surgery
Stony Brook University Medical Center
Stony Brook, NY 11794, USA.

Laurie Kirstein, MD
Assistant Professor, Division of Breast Surgery
Beth Israel Medical Center
New York, NY 10003, USA.

Robert R. Kuske, Jr., MD
Arizona Oncology Services Cancer Research Foundation
8994 East Desert Cove Avenue, Suite 100
Scottsdale, AZ 85260, USA.

Sunny Mitchell, MD
White Plains Hospital
41 East Post Road
White Plains, NY 10601, USA.

Monica Morrow, MD
Chief, Breast Service, Department of Surgery
Memorial Sloan-Kettering Cancer Center
New York, NY 10065, USA.

Suri Ponamgi, MD
Fort Lee Plastic Surgery
Fort Lee, NJ 07024, USA.

Christine H. Rohde, MD
Assistant Professor of Clinical Surgery
Division of Plastic Surgery
New York-Presbyterian Hospital/Columbia
New York, NY, USA.

Walter Paul Weber, MD
Breast Service, Department of Surgery
Memorial Sloan-Kettering Cancer Center
New York, NY 10065, USA.
Department of General Surgery
University Hospital of Basel
Basel, Switzerland.

# ACKNOWLEDGMENTS

I would like to thank Shan-san Wu, MSKCC, for his editorial assistance, and Anne Erickson, Certified Medical Illustrator at Gnumedia, for her artwork.

# INTRODUCTION

Oncoplastic surgery is becoming a discussion-generating topic in the field of breast cancer surgery. There are, however, no parameters to clearly define what is meant by the term "oncoplastic surgery." Some believe that oncoplastic surgery translates into larger resection of primary cancer with "better" margins while simultaneously using plastic surgical techniques to repair the defects created. Others define it as a combination of two surgical disciplines: surgical oncology and plastic surgery.

When a patient presents with breast cancer to my office, I have three priorities in mind: patient survival, local control of the disease, and quality of life. I have listed these priorities by their order of importance. Breast conservation is as effective as mastectomy in survival, and perhaps in local control of breast cancer. It is currently performed in more than 60% of cases with stage I and II disease.

Breast conservation seems to carry a better quality of life due to the fact that the organ is preserved. It is intuitive, however, that the final cosmetic result following resection of the cancer and radiation therapy will impact quality of life and patient recovery. In modern societies, fashionable clothing frequently molds to or exposes a significant part of the breast. Furthermore, in Europe, it is becoming more customary to appear topless on the beach; hence the importance of maintaining a cosmetically appealing breast following breast-conservation therapy.

What we present in this textbook is our perception of oncoplastic breast surgery: to resect the breast cancer in an oncologically sound manner while maintaining — or perhaps enhancing — the cosmetic appearance of the breast. Oncologically sound principles do not necessarily mean wider margins and larger resections. We have dedicated a chapter to presenting an evidence-based definition of adequate margins.

We have divided oncoplastic approaches into two broad categories: simple and complex. These categories are not etched in stone; there is some crossover between the two. Simple oncoplastic procedures fall into the category of when the tumor is small and when excision of such lesions may require removal of less than 25% of the breast. The complex procedures usually fall into the category of when the tumors are relatively large compared with the size of the breast. Resection of relatively large tumors may necessitate excision of large volume, defined as greater than 25%, of the breast, with significant rearrangement of the tissue as part of a mastopexy or breast-reductive procedure. We believe that breast and general surgeons will be able to immediately implement all of the simple, and some of the complex, oncoplastic techniques described in this book. The more complex oncoplastic techniques will require specialized training or consultation with a plastic surgeon. We strongly encourage approaching the more complex oncoplastic procedures with a team composed of a general/breast/oncologic surgeon, and a plastic surgeon who is well versed in such procedures.

The main purpose of this book is to detail the basic principles and techniques of oncoplastic procedures, and to attempt to elucidate the evidence underpinning such procedures. We believe that the sound application of oncoplastic techniques requires a fundamental understanding of breast anatomy; basic breast measurements are presented here in separate chapters.

Neoadjuvant therapy appears to be helpful in achieving a better cosmetic result, and we have dedicated a chapter to discussing its implementation relative to oncoplastic techniques. We also address skin and nipple sparing mastectomies in two separate chapters as these techniques may enhance the final reconstructive result following mastectomy. These chapters may be reviewed independently. It is, however, preferable to refer to them that way after completing the book as a whole.

This book is directed to the general surgeon and the breast surgeon, as well as to the plastic surgeons who will collaborate in these interventions. It is my wish that this book will widen your horizons and enhance your patients' satisfaction.

# Chapter 1

# SURGICAL ANATOMY OF THE BREAST

Mahmoud El-Tamer* and Sunny Mitchell†

*Breast Service, Department of Surgery,
Memorial Sloan-Kettering Cancer Center,
New York, NY 10065, USA*

† *Women's Breast Center, Department of Surgery,
Tully Health Center,
Stamford, CT 06902, USA*

## 1.1 Topology of the Breast: An Overview

The breasts are the most superficial aspect of the anterior chest wall. The skin immediately over the breast tissue is characterized with a nipple areola complex (NAC), centrally located in young adults. The borders of the breast are the second intercostal space superiorly, the midaxillary line laterally, the inframammary line inferiorly, and the sternum medially. The breast overlies the pectoralis major muscle and part of the serratus anterior, external oblique, and rectus abdominus. The NAC is generally located in the fourth and fifth intercostal spaces in males and prepubescent children.

Many studies have reported that women's breasts are more frequently asymmetric.[1,2] In a recent study, Avsar *et al.* measured anthropometric breast values in 386 female students and reported symmetric breast volume in only 35% of subjects.[3] Multiple studies have been done over the years on all aspects of breast anatomy, including arterial supply, venous drainage, and lymphatic patterns. Discrepancies have existed in the published literature in aspects such as lymphatic mapping, dominant arterial supplies, and general vascular patterns. Information presented in the following paragraphs represents the most current research and findings. Along with the currently supported theories, we have also listed papers of historical precedence which are of interest and relevance to all surgeons.

## 1.2 Fascia

The breast is enveloped by a pseudofascial plane: the superficial fascia of the anterior thoracic wall. This fascia splits into an anterior and a posterior layer. The posterior or deep layer of the superficial fascia is found deep posterior to the breast tissue, overlying the retromammary space and pectoralis muscle fascia. The retromammary bursa is a distinct space between the posterior fascia of the breast and the pectoralis fascia, which facilitates mobility of the breast over the chest wall. The superficial fascia joins the cervical fascia at the level of the second intercostal space and superficial abdominal fascia of Camper after the inframammary line. The anterior border of the breast is thought to lie in the subdermal plane.[4]

## 1.3 Raising Flaps

The identification of the appropriate plane is crucial when creating flaps for breast-conservation surgery or mastectomy. Immediately below the skin lies the subdermal system, the subcutaneous tissue, and, finally, the breast parenchyma (Figure 1.1).[4] A dissection in between the subdermal and subcutaneous system results in excision of all breast tissue and preservation of adequately perfused flaps (Figure 1.1, Plane 1). While raising flaps for the repair of the defect, we recommend that flaps be raised between the subcutaneous tissue and the breast (Figure 1.1, Plane 2).

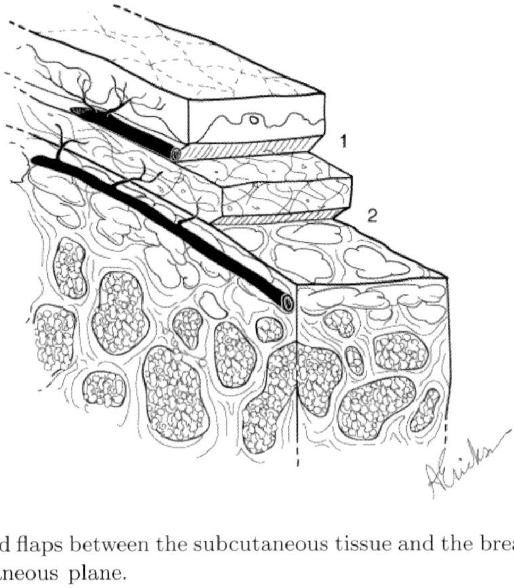


Figure 1.1. Raised flaps between the subcutaneous tissue and the breast. (1) Subdermal plane. (2) Subcutaneous plane.

When utilizing tumescent injection and sharp dissection for creating flaps, the tumescent solution is injected into the subcutaneous space, and dissection proceeds between the subcutaneous space and the subdermal system. Flap thickness varies between patients. In the same patient, the thickness of the flaps varies in different locations. Blood loss is minimal when surgeons use the appropriate plane because the connecting vessels between the breast and the subdermal tissue are miniscule.

## 1.4 Ligaments of Cooper and Horizontal Septum

The deep and superficial layers of the superficial fascia are linked through fibrous bands, known as ligaments of Cooper. These ligaments originate from the pectoralis fascia at the level of the fifth rib and extend into the overlying skin as well as the pectoralis major muscle, dividing the breast tissue into septae and aiding in suspending the breast to the chest wall.[5,6]

A ligamentous septum comprising a horizontal fibrous septum originating from the pectoralis fascia at the level of the fifth rib and its vertical ligamentous suspension provides medial and lateral lines of fixation on either side of the breast.[5] This also gives rise to a superficial aspect that merges into the overlying skin.[5] The medial superficial ligament is thought to be weaker and stretches into the skin overlying the sternum. The lateral stronger superficial ligament creates a strong connection between the pectoralis minor as well as the skin and overlying fascia of the axilla along the midaxillary line, producing the axillary hollow.[5] The superficial part of the horizontal septum is a thickening of the ligaments of Cooper, stretching for the same origin at the level of the fifth rib to the inframammary line.[5] The horizontal ligamentous septum guides the neurovascular supply of the breast and nipple areola complex. Varying degrees of ptosis are a direct reflection of the laxity of the ligaments of Cooper.

Between the breast and the pectoralis major fascia exists the space known as the retromammary bursa, which facilitates the mobility of the breast on the chest wall. Adhering to this space while raising local flaps for breast-conservation surgery is crucial to the viability of tne breast tissue; it will preserve the integrity of the neurovascular supply to the breast tissue, and minimize fat and tissue necrosis, particularly in older women with fatty breasts.

## 1.5 Arterial Supply of the Breast

Salmon developed a successful injection technique in cadavers that allowed him to delineate the arterial supply of the breast in fine detail.[7] He

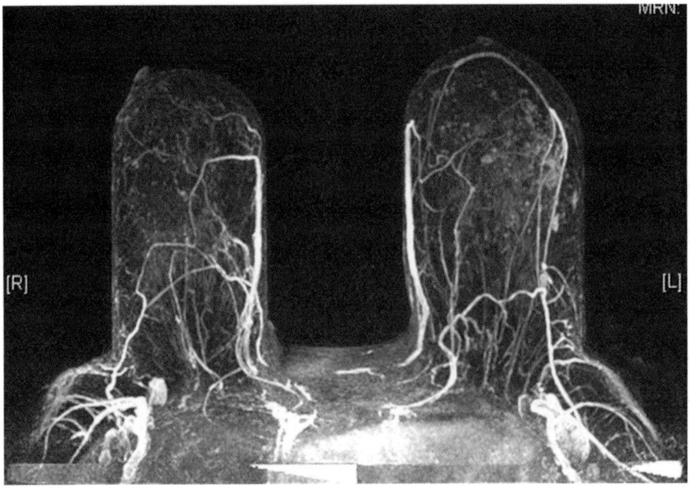


Figure 1.2. MRI reconstruction of the blood supply of the breast. (Courtesy of Dr. Jennifer Kaplan, Memorial Sloan-Kettering Cancer Center, New York, NY.)

found that the blood supply to the breast originated from 3 systems, the axillary, internal mammary, and intercostals, which are more commonly known today as the lateral mammary, internal mammary, and intercostal branches. The predominant vascular supply of the breast is from the internal mammary, anterior intercostal, lateral thoracic, and thoracoacromial arteries.[8] The inferior and central pedicles of the breast were thought to be hypovascularized.[9] This idea was challenged by Salmon, who attributed this misconception to an inadequate injection technique. He has proposed that the inferior and central portions of the breast receive arterial supply from perforators through the pectoralis muscle. These perforators are well visualized during a mastectomy while taking the breast off the pectoralis major muscle. Figure 1.2 represents a magnetic resonance imaging (MRI) reconstruction of the blood supply of the breast, clearly showing the lateral mammary, internal mammary, and intercostal perforators.

### 1.5.1 *Lateral Mammary Artery*

This artery supplies the lateral aspect of the breast; it is a direct branch of the axillary artery or one of its tributaries.[10] Salmon has observed the lateral mammary artery to arise from the external mammary artery, lateral thoracic artery, or directly from the axillary artery.[7] Occasionally, it is referred to as the lateral thoracic artery, which is thought to be incorrect as the lateral thoracic artery supplies the lateral upper chest wall. The lateral mammary artery enters the breast over the axillary tail laterally at the

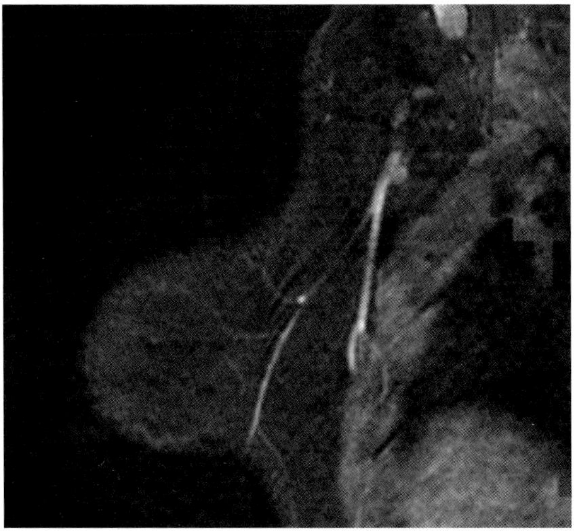

Figure 1.3. Lateral mammary artery, traveling through the breast.

level of the third or fourth rib. The artery runs superficially and takes an anterolateral course, sending branches into the breast tissue, the overlying skin, and the chest wall. This artery consistently contributes deep subcutaneous branches to the NAC[6] and has been cited as contributing 30% of the blood flow to the breast.[11] The branches of the lateral mammary artery travel diagonally in a medial direction until fading beyond the lateral aspect of the inframammary line (Figure 1.3). The lateral mammary artery connects with the medial artery around the NAC either through the superficial or posterior branches (Figure 1.2).

The lateral mammary artery is pivotal for the survival of the laterally based breast reduction. This artery may frequently be ligated during an axillary node dissection. When planning an oncoplastic procedure in a patient who is undergoing an axillary node dissection, one has to avoid mammaplasties that are laterally based.

### 1.5.2 *Internal Mammary Artery*

The internal mammary artery (internal thoracic artery) originates from the subclavian artery, traveling parallel and posterior to the lateral border of the sternum. This artery provides up to 60% of the blood supply to the breast, mostly the medial portion. It sends anterior and posterior perforating branches through the parasternal and intercostal spaces. The largest branches perforate through one of the first few intercostal spaces. The anterior perforators arise from the first 4 intercostal spaces,

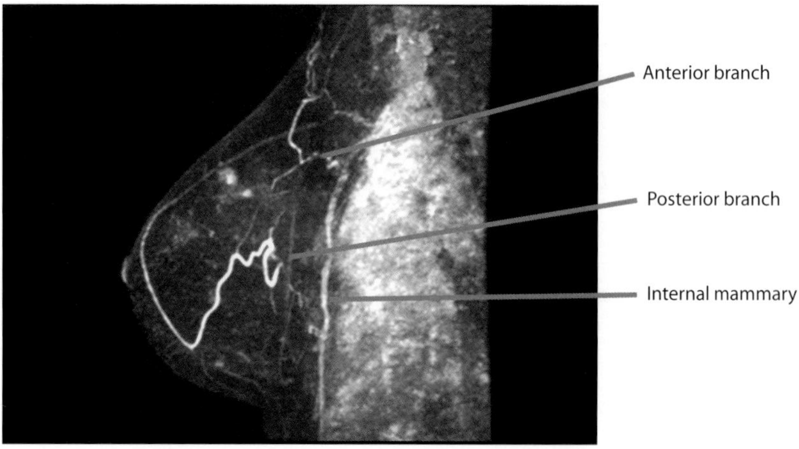


Figure 1.4. MRI reconstitution of the branches of the internal mammary, showing the anterior and the posterior branches. (Courtesy of Dr. Jennifer Kaplan, Memorial Sloan-Kettering Cancer Center, New York, NY.)

just medial to the sternum. Perforators from the second and third intercostal spaces are the most consistent, while those from the first and fourth are not as common.[12] These anterior perforators split into cutaneous and breast branches (Figure 1.2). Preserving the integrity of the cutaneous branches is crucial when performing a skin-sparing or nipple areola-sparing mastectomy.

The posterior medial perforators of the internal thoracic artery (only described by Salmon) arise more laterally from the intercostal spaces through the pectoralis fascia into the breast and supply the deep portion of the breast tissue. These vessels appear to be branches of the internal thoracic artery, emerging from the fourth and fifth intercostal spaces. These vessels may have been reported by others and referred to as branches of the intercostals. Figure 1.4 is an MRI reconstitution of the branches of the internal mammary, showing the anterior and the posterior branches. This blood supply supports a significant portion of the medial aspect of the breast as well as the NAC. This is the main blood supply for medially based breast reduction. The posterior medial mammary arteries are important contributors to the arterial blood supply of the inferiorly based breast reduction pedicle.

### 1.5.3 *Thoracoacromial Artery*

The pectoral branch of the thoracoacromial artery is a less-important blood supply source to the breast. It is located between the pectoralis major and minor muscles, entering the subcutaneous breast tissue at the deltopectoral groove.[6] Branches may reach the posterior aspect of the breast as well as be accompanied by lymphatics that may allow for metastasis to Rotter's nodes.

### 1.5.4 *Posterior Intercostal Arteries*

The posterior intercostal arteries give off branches that perforate the chest wall and run laterally to the pectoral muscle, giving rise to vessels that supply the lower outer quadrant of the breast. The contribution of these vessels has been debated.

## 1.6 Venous Drainage of the Breast

Blood drains from the breast through a superficial and deep system. The medial segment of the breast was found to have a superficial drainage pattern, whereas the lateral venous drainage was found to run deeper.[8] The dominant drainage pattern of the breast has been found to be superficial. The subareolar plexus radiates most frequently to the superomedial and inferior pole.[13,14] The dominant drainage route was found to be via the third and fourth intercostal spaces.[13,14] Superomedial drainage is via the second and third intercostal spaces, while lower pole drainage is via the fourth and fifth intercostal spaces.[13,14] The subareolar plexus has been found consistently in the subcutaneous plane.[13] The nipple venous drainage appears to run medially to the internal mammary veins.

Venous insufficiency is often the culprit for vascular compromise in breast-reduction surgery. An important point to remember is that when the lateral veins are divided, the venous drainage of the NAC becomes dependent on the superficial veins in the superomedial pedicle.[8] Additional studies on breast vasculature are included.[7,10–12,15,16] These studies are interesting and include results commonly found today, along with multiple discrepancies, including currently unrecognized vessels.

## 1.7 Lymphatics

The axilla is accepted as the main basin for lymphatic drainage of the breast. Whether lymphatics drain into the subareolar complex prior to traveling to the axilla is yet to be confirmed. Suami *et al.*,[17] through radiologic lymph injection into cadavers, summarized the following:

(1) No difference was found in superficial lymph vasculature between males and females.

(2) The midaxillary line divides the lymph territories of the upper torso.
(3) A sentinel node of the upper limb also covers a wide range of the anterior upper torso.
(4) The lymph-collecting vessels from the nipple merge with the vessels from the lower part of the torso before reaching the axilla.
(5) In the female breast, some torso lymph vessels run through the breast tissue.

## 1.8 Nerve Supply

Initially described in detail by Sir Astley Cooper in 1840, the breast has since been consistently found to be innervated from the lateral and anterior cutaneous branches of the second to sixth intercostal nerves.[18,19] The lateral branches pierce the chest wall musculature at the midaxillary line and travel medially. These nerves divide into a superficial branch and a deep branch at the edge of the pectoral muscle (Figure 1.5).

The superficial branch travels subcutaneously, whereas the deep branches travel along the pectoralis fascia for a few centimeters and then merge through the breast tissue to the surface at the midclavicular line.

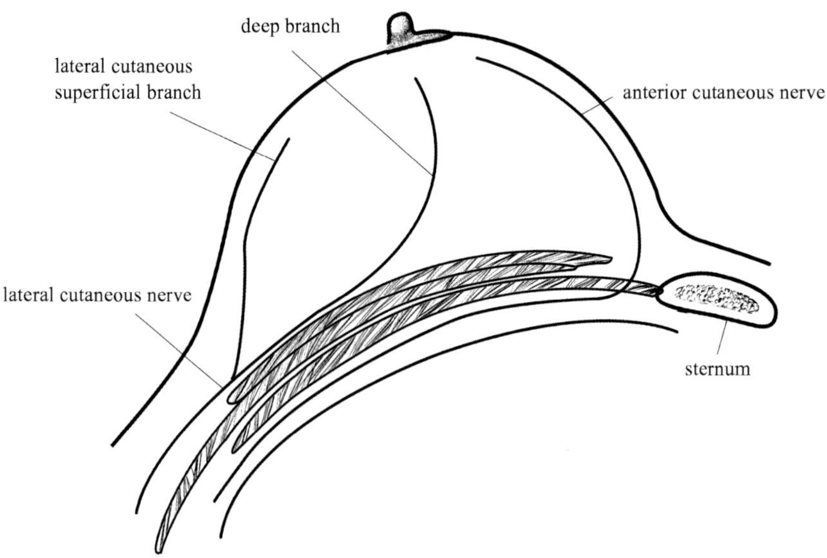


Figure 1.5. Nerve supply to the breast. The lateral cutaneous nerve divides into superficial and deep branches.

The anterior cutaneous branches merge through the chest wall at the edge of the sternum and travel superficially toward the nipple, thereby supplying the medial aspect of the breast.

The NAC innervation is not consistent, hence the controversy. It is agreed upon, however, that the innervation of the NAC is from the anterior and lateral branches of the third to fifth intercostal nerves. The fourth lateral cutaneous nerve is the most frequent source of sensation to the NAC, mostly via its deep branches.

Hamdi and colleagues have reported that in 93% of breasts, the deep branch of the lateral cutaneous nerve innervates the nipple. As previously described, the deep branch runs within the pectoralis fascia, curves straight up through the glandular tissue at the level of the midclavicular line, and sends its terminal branches straight to the nipple.[20]

The third, fourth, and fifth anterior branches innervate the medial aspect of the NAC. The nerves enter the NAC superficially at its medial edge, mostly between 8:00 o′clock and 11:00 o′clock for the left breast and 1:00 o′clock to 4:00 o′clock for the right breast. When planning a terminal duct excision or removing a centrally located tumor, we strongly recommend avoiding a medial periareolar incision because it will interrupt the anterior cutaneous branches that will be the only innervation to the NAC. Understanding the innervation of the NAC is important in planning incisions and access for resection of a tumor. Historical papers on breast innervation are included.[21,22]

## 1.9 Nipple Areola Complex

### 1.9.1 *Innervation*

Innervation of the NAC is derived from the anterior and lateral cutaneous branches of the second to fourth intercostal nerves. The fourth lateral and medial intercostal (anterior cutaneous) branches provide the most consistent innervation (see Section 1.8).[14,23]

### 1.9.2 *Blood Supply*

The NAC's most consistent blood supply source is medial via the internal thoracic artery.[4,6,24] The NAC is also supplied with blood from the anterior intercostal arteries as well as the lateral thoracic artery. Very rarely do direct branches of the axillary artery or posterior intercostal arteries supply the NAC.[4,24] This is of clinical relevance in understanding how to work within the confines of the most likely patterns of arterial supply to the NAC. For the most part, NAC venous drainage appears to run medially to the internal mammary veins.[8]

### 1.9.3 *Areola*

The areola contains Montgomery glands. These are sebaceous glands, capable of secreting milk. The Morgagni tubercles are small, raised papules on the areola through which Montgomery glands have egress.[25]

The NAC is an important landmark of the breast. Its position and potential repositioning is of utmost importance in breast-conserving surgery as well as nipple-sparing mastectomy. A periareolar incision of half or less than half the circumference of the NAC is thought to be well tolerated, resulting in minimal chance of epidermolysis. When utilizing oncoplastic techniques, it is often necessary to reposition the NAC by de-epithelializing the periareolar skin (as in the Benelli mastopexy). The NAC is dependent on the lateral or medial dermal vasculature and underlying parenchyma for blood supply.

Maintaining a 0.5 to 1.0 cm thickness of glandular tissue under the NAC while raising flaps in breast-conservation cases helps in survival of the NAC.[26] The dermal vasculature is responsible for the blood supply of a de-epithelialized NAC once it is separated from the underlying gland.[26] In an inferior pole mammoplasty, the vascular supply of the NAC is derived from the inferior and posterior glandular tissue. The NAC maintains its blood supply via the superior pedicle after a wide-local excision via a J-mammaplasty or superior pedicle mastopexy.[26]

Operating on the breast is quite forgiving. To achieve excellent cosmetic results after a sound oncologic procedure, a full understanding of the anatomy, with particular emphasis on the blood supply, of the breast and overlying skin is required.

## References

1. Bostwick J. (1983) Correction of breast asymmetries. *Aesthetic and Reconstructive Breast Surgery.* Mosby Company, St. Louis, Toronto, London, p. 252.
2. Smith DJ, Jr., Palin WE, Jr., Katch VL, Bennett JE. (1986) Breast volume and anthropomorphic measurements: Normal values. *Plast Reconstr Surg* 78(3):331–335.
3. Avsar DK, Aygit AC, Benlier E, *et al.* (2010) Anthropometric breast measurement: A study of 385 Turkish female students. *Aesthet Surg J* 30(1): 44–50.
4. Pearl RM, Johnson D. (1983) The vascular supply to the skin: An anatomical and physiological reappraisal — Part II. *Ann Plast Surg* 11(3):196–205.
5. Wueringer E, Tschabitscher M. (2003) New aspects of the topography of the mammary gland regarding its neurovascular supply along a regular ligamentous suspension. *Eur J Morphol* 40(3):181.

6. O'Dey D, Prescher A, Pallua N. (2007) Vascular reliability of nipple-areola complex-bearing pedicles: An anatomical microdissection study. *Plast Reconstr Surg* 119(4):1167–1177.
7. Salmon M. (1939) Les arthres de la glande mammaire. *Ann Anat Pathol* 16: 477–500.
8. Michelle le Roux C, Kiil BJ, Pan WR, *et al.* (2010) Preserving the neurovascular supply in the Hall-Findlay superomedial pedicle breast reduction: An anatomical study. *J Plast Reconstr Aesthet Surg* 63(4): 655–662.
9. Maliniac JW. (1943) Arterial blood supply of the breast. *Arch Surg* 47:329–343.
10. Cunningham L. (1977) The anatomy of the arteries and veins of the breast. *J Surg Oncol* 9(1): 71–85.
11. Nakajima H, Imanishi N, Aiso S. (1995) Arterial anatomy of the nipple-areola complex. *Plast Reconstr Surg* 96(4):843–845.
12. Palmer JH, Taylor GI. (1986) The vascular territories of the anterior chest wall. *Br J Plast Surg* 39(3):287–299.
13. Corduff N, Rozen WM, Taylor GI. (2010) The superficial venous drainage of the breast: A clinical study and implications for breast reduction surgery. *J Plast Reconstr Aesthet Surg* 63(5):809–813.
14. Jaspars JJ, Posma AN, van Immerseel AA, Gittenberger-de Groot AC. (1997) The cutaneous innervation of the female breast and nipple-areola complex: Implications for surgery. *Br J Plast Surg* 50(4):249–259.
15. Anson BJ, Wright RR, Wolfer JH. (1939) Blood supply of the mammary gland. *Surg Gynecol Obstet* 69:468–473.
16. Wuringer E, Mader N, Posch E, Holle J. (1998) Nerve and vessel supplying ligamentous suspension of the mammary gland. *Plast Reconstr Surg* 101(6):1486–1493.
17. Suami H, O'Neill JK, Pan WR, Taylor GI. (2008) Superficial lymphatic system of the upper torso: Preliminary radiographic results in human cadavers. *Plast Reconstr Surg* 121(4):1231–1239.
18. Sarhadi NS, Shaw Dunn J, Lee FD, Soutar DS. (1996) An anatomical study of the nerve supply of the breast, including the nipple and areola. *Br J Plast Surg* 49(3):156–164.
19. Sarhadi NS, Shaw-Dunn J, Soutar DS. (1997) Nerve supply of the breast with special reference to the nipple and areola: Sir Astley Cooper revisited. *Clin Anat* 10(4):283–288.
20. Hamdi M, Wurenger E, Schlenz I, Kuzbari R. (2005) Anatomy of the breast: A clinical application. In: Hamdi M, Hammond DC, Nahai F (eds.), *Vertical Scar Mammaplasty*, Springer Verlag, Berlin, p. 6.
21. Craig RD, Sykes PA. (1970) Nipple sensitivity following reduction mammaplasty. *Br J Plast Surg* 23(2):165–172.
22. Regnault P. (1974) Reduction mammaplasty by the "B" technique. *Plast Reconstr Surg* 53(1):19–24.
23. Schlenz I, Kuzbari R, Gruber H, Holle J. (2000) The sensitivity of the nipple-areola complex: An anatomic study. *Plast Reconstr Surg* 105(3): 905–909.

24. van Deventer PV. (2004) The blood supply to the nipple-areola complex of the human mammary gland. *Aesthet Plast Surg* 28(6):393–398.
25. Nicholson BT, Harvey JA, Cohen MA. (2009) Nipple-areolar complex: Normal anatomy and benign and malignant processes. *Radiographics* 29(2): 509–523.
26. Clough KB, Kaufman GJ, Nos C, *et al.* (2010) Improving breast cancer surgery: A classification and quadrant per quadrant atlas for oncoplastic surgery. *Ann Surg Oncol* 17(5):1375–1391.

# Chapter 2

# SURGICAL LANDMARKS AND MEASUREMENTS

Suri Ponamgi* and Mahmoud El-Tamer†

**Fort Lee Plastic Surgery, Fort Lee, NJ 07024, USA*

*†Breast Service, Department of Surgery, Memorial Sloan-Kettering Cancer Center, New York, NY 10065, USA*

Preoperative marking is an integral step for a successful outcome in oncoplastic surgery procedures of the breast. Because of the diversity of the female breast physiognomy, accurate and reproducible measurements are difficult to achieve.

The young breast is a conical mound with the nipple and areola at its highest point, which is the center of the mound. As the breast ages and its size increases, it develops ptosis with a downward slant in the upper pole, and descent of the nipple complex on the mound that is dependent on the increase in volume. As the breast goes through the hormonal changes that occur during pregnancy, there is an initial increase in its volume, with eventual deflation and ptosis after childbirth. The breast can also change in size and shape with obesity and weight gain; the fluctuations in volume, associated with weight changes, are seen more in postmenopausal breasts, where most of the breast tissue is replaced by fat.

Surgical treatment for breast cancer has varied greatly, from the most-radical Hagensen mastectomy, to extended radical mastectomy, to the present-day conservative nipple-sparing surgery in select cases. Several papers have focused on how to reconstruct partial mastectomy defects by rearranging the remaining breast tissue and relocating the nipple and areola complex. In many instances, even in autologous tissue or staged-implant reconstructions, the opposite breast must be treated to achieve symmetry. Planning for surgery in such cases must be done simultaneously by marking both breasts at the same time.

## 2.1 Breast Measurement

In the 1950s, Penn defined breast aesthetics by studying 150 healthy women, 20 of whom had "perfect" breasts.[1] He found that an equilateral triangle existed between the suprasternal notch and both nipples in those women whose limbs were approximately 21 cm in length. The distance was also the same from the midclavicular line to the nipple. In Penn's study, the average nipple-to-inframammary–fold distance was 6.9 cm. Although these symmetry findings are not absolutes because patients and their breasts come in all shapes and sizes, they are a useful guide to keep in mind.

Most recently, Westreich published results of anthropometric measurements in 50 women with aesthetically "perfect" breasts.[2] His study cites previously published studies by Penn[1] in 1955 and Smith DJ *et al.*[3] in 1986, and differs from them in that his subjects were women with only "perfect" breasts. His study reported the following norms: (1) the acromial span (obtained by doubling the distance between the acromium and the suprasternal notch) had a mean value of 36.52 cm; (2) the range was between 32 cm in a subject with a 425-cc breast volume and 41 cm in a subject with 325-cc breast volume; (3) the midclavicle-to-nipple distance was 18.6 cm with a range between 16.5 cm (305-cc breast volume) and 23 cm (375-cc breast volume); (4) the mean nipple-to-inframammary–crease distance was 6.95 cm (Figure 2.1); (5) this distance increased with an increase in volume; (6) in inverted "T" breast reductions, this measurement was approximately between 5 cm and 6 cm, depending on the diameter of the reconstructed areola, and the length of the vertical component of the scar did not exceed 5 cm; (7) the mean value of the nipple-to-nipple distance was 19.35 cm; and (8) the suprasternal notch-to-nipple distance was 18.59 cm.

In the clinical setting, wide variations can be seen depending on the attachments of the breast to the chest wall. If such variations are not considered and measurements are made with the assumption that the breasts are in normal position, disastrous results can occur. It is the breast base (the attachment of the breast to the chest wall) that determines the breast's relative position on the chest wall. This issue was studied by Hall-Findley,[4] who found that regardless of suspension technique used in breast reduction and lift surgeries, a low-positioned breast will always remain low, and that to achieve upper-pole fullness in these breasts, one may have to resort to using an implant. She also suggests that a safer way to determine the new position for the nipple in a low-positioned breast is to locate the upper pole of the breast on the chest wall and position the upper pole of the new areola at 8 cm from this point, inferiorly along the nipple meridian. To avoid bottoming-out, most breast tissue that is removed should be from the lower pole. In a markedly ptotic breast, it may even be appropriate to reduce the breast in the lower pole during mastopexy and add an implant for volume if upper-pole fullness is desired. According to the observations of Westreich, a high-positioned breast needs a smaller volume to appear adequate whereas, in a low-positioned breast, a larger breast volume may be appropriate.

In the oncoplastic setting, the shape, size, and location of the defect are clearly dictated by the location and size of the primary. The surgical team will have to plan the nipple repositioning, based on the oncologic procedure. The mean inframammary-crease length has a high correlation with the breast volume. In reduction patients with large pendulous breasts, there is an extension of this fold laterally, resulting in dog-ears and extension of the submammary scars laterally, with need for liposuction of the folds. In the vertical technique, mere liposuction of the folds will improve the contour.

Westreich *et al.* also observed areola shape and size in their study, reporting that 52% of the women studied had symmetrically round areolas, and that areola size increased with the size of the breast. The most attractive areolar diameter is approximately 35–45 mm, and the ideal nipple projection is usually 4–7 mm.[5]

To achieve good results in breast surgery, there is still no substitute for adequate preoperative evaluation, experience, and surgical skill. A cookbook technique, based only on measurements, will not suit all patients. Preoperative planning with a rough estimate of the size and location of the defect, and good aesthetic sense with the ability to modify if necessary during surgery, will reduce complications and yield better results. As a result, the importance of an adequate review of all breast images and appropriate discussion with all members of the surgical team is crucial.

## 2.2 Breast Markings

Measurements and breast markings should be made with the woman standing in the normal anatomic position, with the shoulders back, head facing straight ahead, and arms alongside. First, the fixed landmarks are identified: the sternal notch; the clavicle; the midline; and the nipple meridian (Figure 2.1). The nipple meridian is a vertical line that starts from a point on the clavicle located 6–7 cm lateral to the midsternal notch. The line drops down through the center of the nipple (Figure 2.2, Picture 1). The inframammary lines are then identified on both sides. The surgeon must pay particular attention to the level of the inframammary lines and their symmetry on both sides. The surgeon must make every effort to keep the final position of the nipple along the nipple meridian and at a distance of approximately 19 cm to 22 cm from the midclavicular line.

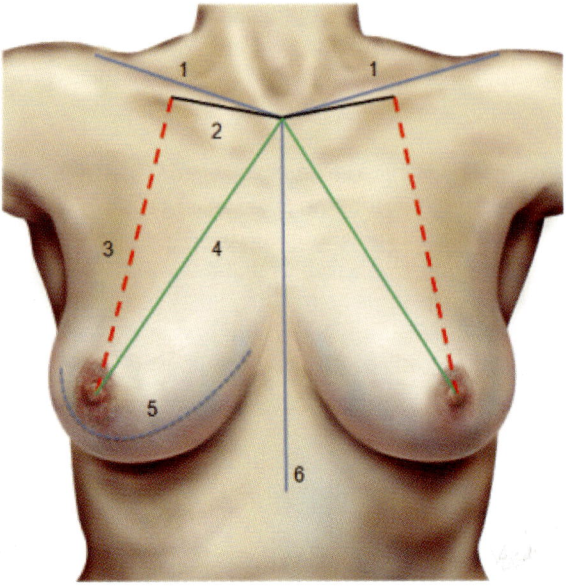


Figure 2.1. Breast landmarks: (1) Acromial span. (2) Sternal-notch nipple meridian (6–7 cm). (3) Nipple meridian. (4) Sternal-notch nipple. (5) Anteriorly transposed inframammary line. (6) Midline.

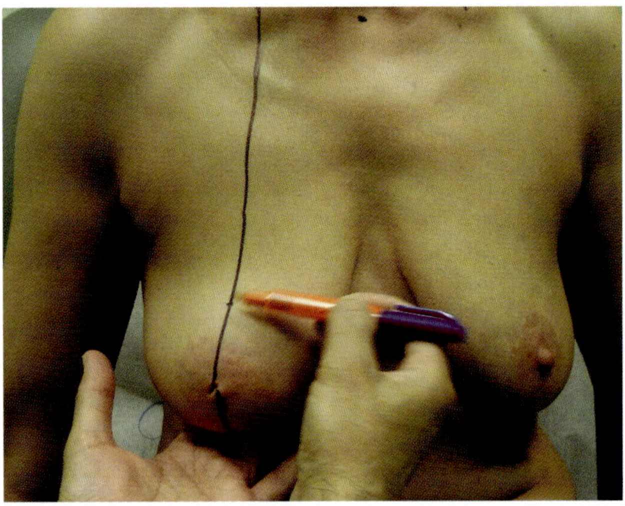

Figure 2.2, Picture 1. A vertical line that starts from a point on the clavicle located 6–7 cm lateral to the midsternal notch. The line drops down through the center of the nipple.

When a mastopexy or a breast reduction is considered as part of the oncoplastic procedure, the markings for the final skin envelope vary depending on the type of reduction, resection, or lift that is planned. The nipple-meridian marking is extended across the inframammary line. The most classical approach has been the Wise pattern or inverted-T mastopexy/reduction. The new position of the nipple must be identified, as well as the amount of skin to be excised or de-epithelialized. The location for the future position of the nipple is marked along the nipple meridian. The inframammary fold is transposed anteriorly on the breast along the nipple meridian to mark the new position for the nipple. The new nipple position will be at the intersection of the inframammary line and the nipple meridian. This is done by placing 4 fingers of the hand behind the breast in the fold and the thumb anteriorly, grasping the breast, and marking the point of the fold transposed anteriorly (Figure 2.2, Picture 2).

In larger breasts, one hand is placed behind at the fold and the other hand is used to palpate the level of the fold on the anterior aspect of the breast.

The position of the nipples is marked symmetrically along the nipple meridian, equidistant from the supra-sternal notch at the highest point of the breast projection on both sides (Figure 2.2, Picture 3, Picture 4).

Marking nipple position using static measurements for reduction or mastopexy incurs the risk of dislocation of the nipple by 1.0–1.5 cm. Nipples placed high or pointing upward may be visible in the cleavage line and appear unaesthetic. A nipple placed low and laterally can be easily

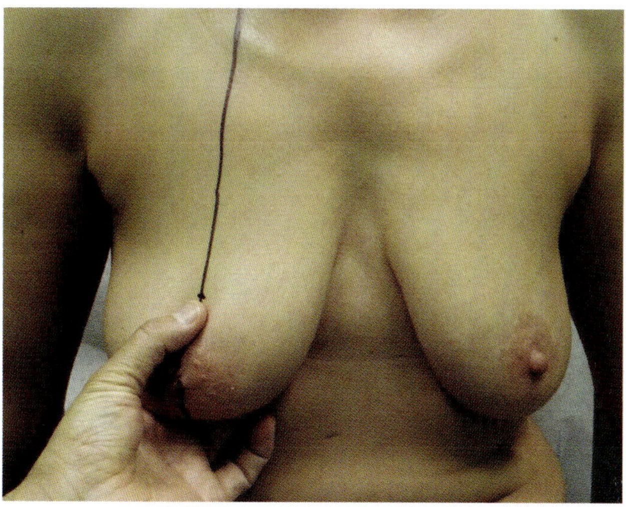

Figure 2.2, Picture 2. Transposing the inframammary fold anteriorly along the nipple meridian to mark the new position for the nipple.

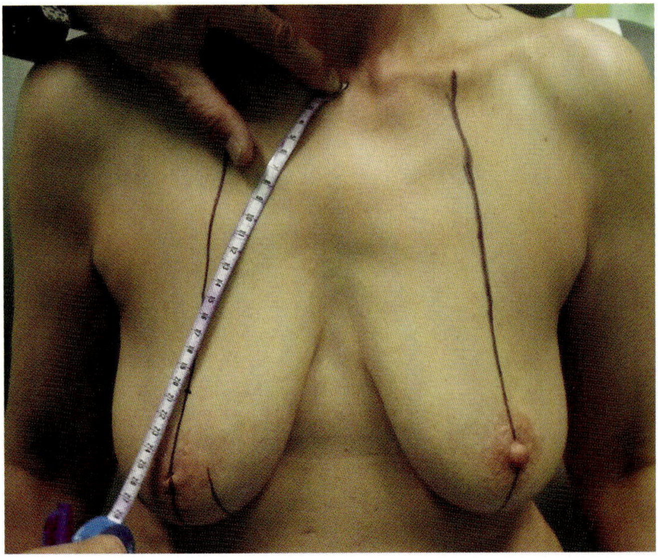

Figure 2.2, Picture 3. Marking the nipple symmetrically along the nipple meridian, equidistant from the supra-sternal notch at the highest point of the breast projection on both sides.

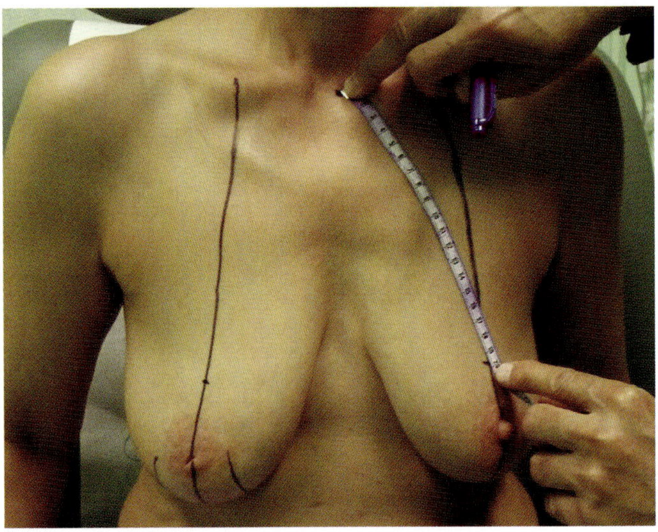

Figure 2.2, Picture 4. Marking the nipple symmetrically along the nipple meridian, equidistant from the supra-sternal notch at the highest point of the breast projection on both sides.

repositioned. A nipple placed high and medially, however, requires more complex procedures with visible scarring. Most techniques mark the height of the nipple along the nipple meridian measuring from anatomical fixed points. We feel that positioning the nipple at 19–22 cm from the midclavicle will be safe. We recommend that surgeons who are novices place the upper edge of the areola at the point of the new nipple.

From the new position of the nipple, a circle with a radius of 2 cm may be marked to receive the areola; alternatively, this can be done after the breast is shaped. The new top of the areola is identified 1.5–2.0 cm superior to the new nipple. Freehand marking is widely used by most surgeons, and requires experience and practice to achieve the desired shape. Imbricating the breast parenchyma or the skin allows surgeons to estimate the amount of skin to be removed in order to reshape the breast with adequate skin tone and tension at the suture lines. Using parenchymal imbrication, the medial and lateral limbs of the vertical ellipse are marked on either side of the areolar complex (Figure 2.2, Picture 5, Picture 6).

The vertical limbs of the Wise pattern extend 7 cm from the position of the future nipple inferomedially and inferolaterally. The nipple meridian marking is extended across the inframammary line to marking point D (Figure 2.2, Picture 7) where the end of vertical limbs will be positioned (points B and C). The medial and lateral ends of the inframammary fold are joined to the end of the vertical limbs, completing the Wise keyhole pattern (Figure 2.2, Picture 7, Picture 8).

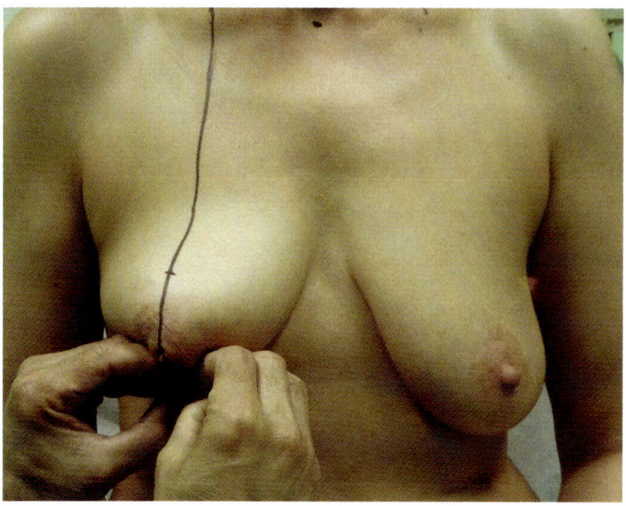

Figure 2.2, Picture 5. Using parenchymal imbrication, the medial and lateral limbs of the vertical ellipse are marked on either side of the areolar complex.

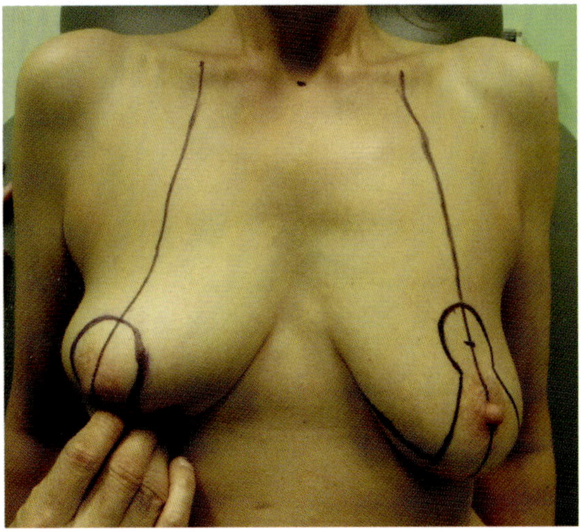

Figure 2.2, Picture 6. Using parenchymal imbrication, the medial and lateral limbs of the vertical ellipse are marked on either side of the areolar complex.

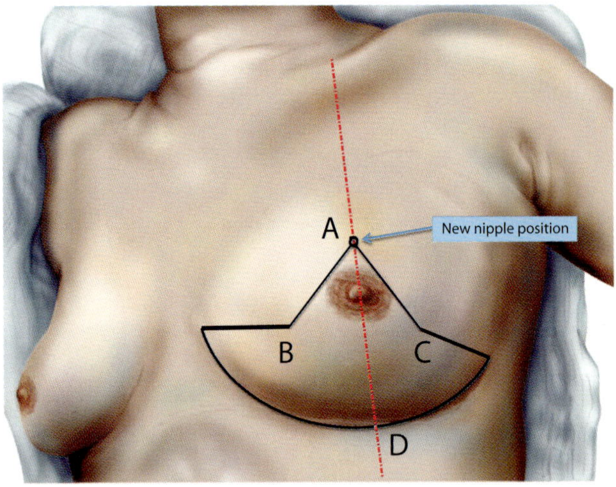


Figure 2.2, Picture 7. The Wise pattern. Points B, C, and D will be sutured together when completing the reshaping of the breast.

Multiple devices are available to facilitate the marking of the breast (Figure 2.2, Picture 9, Picture 10). The standard pattern consisting of a keyhole and a fixed angle of divergence of 110 degrees was modified by McKissock to allow for adjustment of the angle for breasts of varying shapes

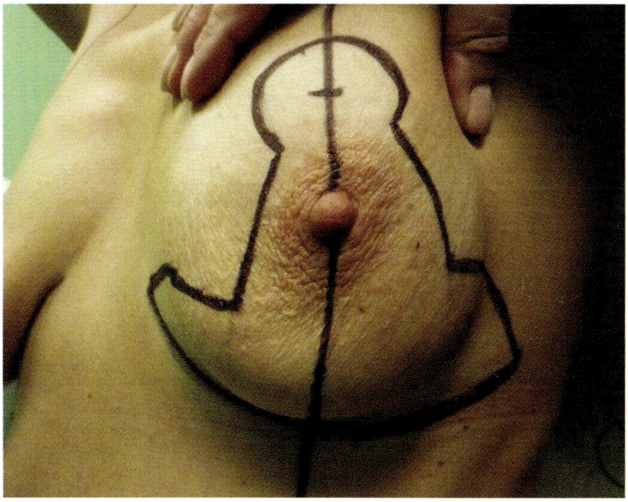

Figure 2.2, Picture 8. Joining of the medial and lateral ends of the inframammary fold to the end of the vertical limbs, completing the Wise keyhole pattern.

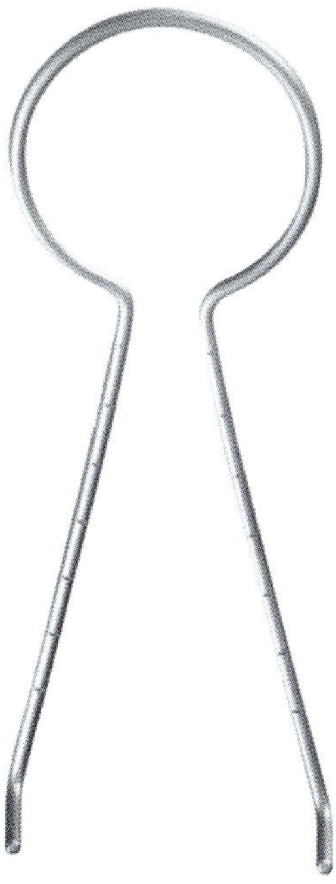

Figure 2.2, Picture 9. McKissock Breast Marker. Miltex Instruments. Available in 38 mm, 42 mm, and 45 mm keyhole diameters.

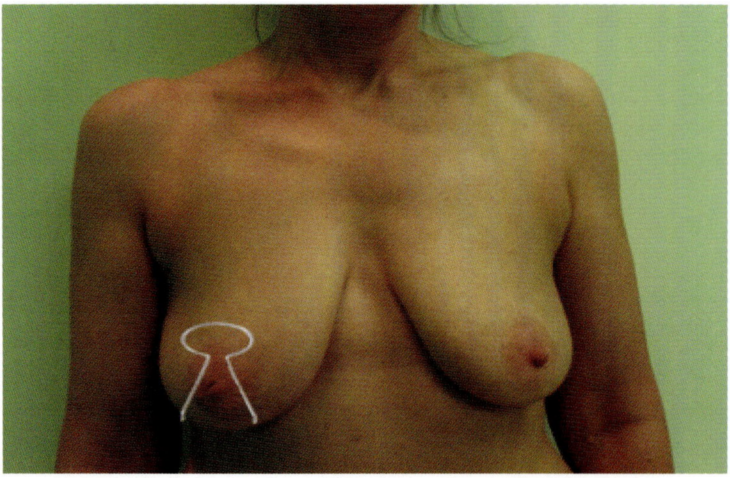

Figure 2.2, Picture 10. Visual application of the McKissock Breast Marker.

and sizes. The lower border of the areola should be at least 5 cm from the final inframammary line.

## 2.3 Vertical Mastopexy/Reduction Markings

The vertical mastopexy/reduction has gained popularity among surgeons as these techniques have eliminated inframammary scars and given greater projection to the breast with higher nipple appearance, especially after the breast settles. In a vertical mastopexy/reduction, the inframammary fold is transposed anteriorly onto the breast, and this point is marked as the highest point of the areola and the nipple positioned 2 cm lower. Compared to the Wise pattern, in the vertical mastopexy, the nipple is placed 1.5–2.0 cm lower; the upper edge of the areola is placed at the intersection of the inframammary line and the nipple meridian. The nipple meridian marking is extended across the inframammary line to the abdominal wall. The vertical ellipse is marked by displacing the breast medially and laterally across the nipple meridian, assessing the horizontal excess of the skin to be removed (Figure 2.2, Picture 11, Picture 12).

At the upper end of the ellipse, a "mosque" or "dome" pattern is marked to inset the future areola, and the 2 vertical limbs of the ellipse are drawn around the areola, stopping 2 cm short of the inframammary fold marking in smaller breasts and 4 cm short of the inframammary-fold marking in larger breasts (Figure 2.2, Picture 13; Figure 2.3). After the markings are completed, they are checked for symmetry, allowing for breast size

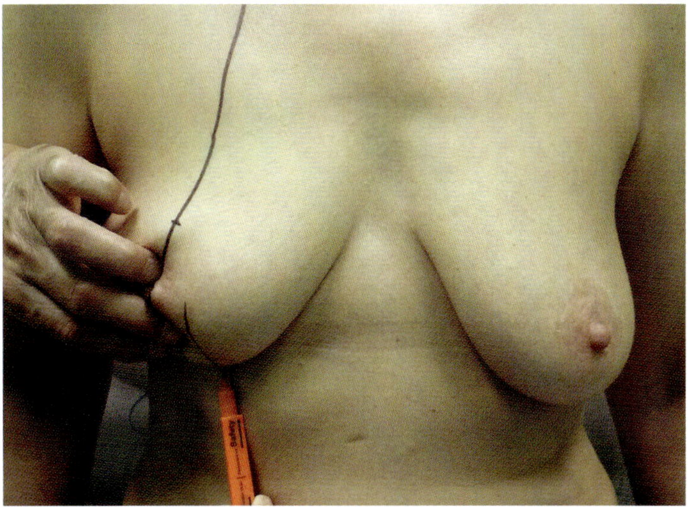

Figure 2.2, Picture 11. Marking of the medial vertical limb by displacing the breast laterally and drawing a line that meets the extension of the nipple meridian on the abdominal wall.

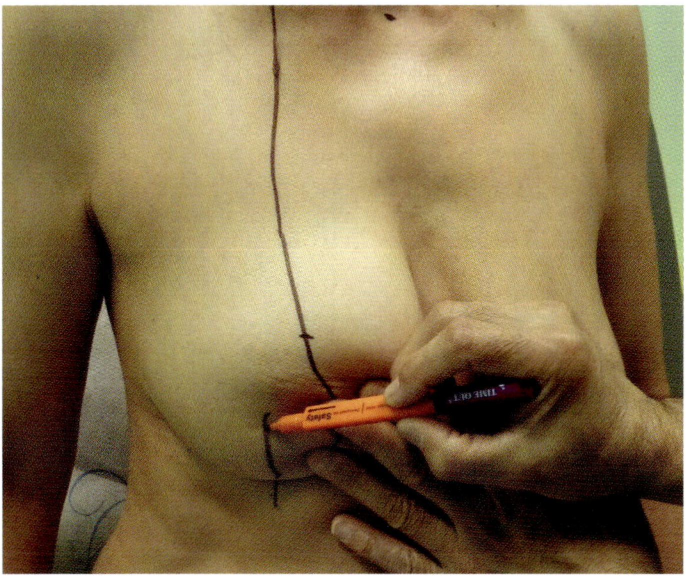

Figure 2.2, Picture 12. Marking the vertical ellipse by displacing the breast medially in a similar fashion to the medial limb.

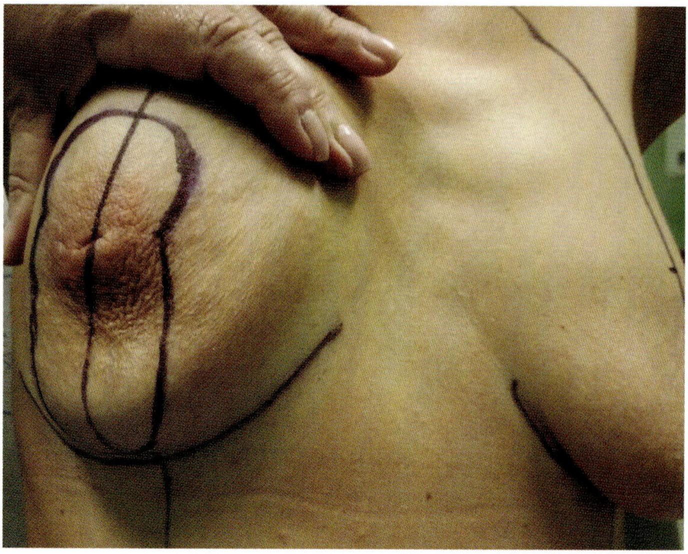

Figure 2.2, Picture 13. "Mosque" or "dome" pattern.

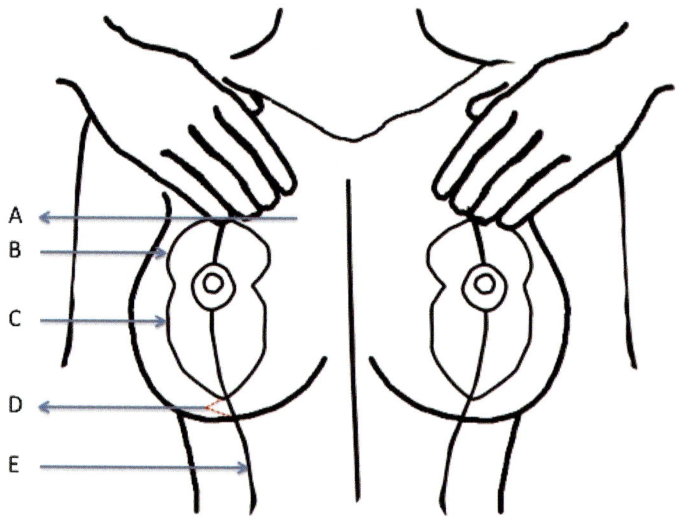


Figure 2.3. Markings for Vertical Reduction. (A) Upper pole of the breast. (B) "Mosque" pattern for areola. (C) Vertical ellipse of skin reduction. (D) Distance from lower pole of vertical ellipse to inframammary crease (2 cm for small breasts and 4 cm for large breasts). (E) Extension of nipple meridian across the inframammary crease.

discrepancy. By imbricating the parenchyma and the skin, the width of the vertical ellipse can be adjusted to avoid tension along the suture line at closure. After breast shaping is completed, the areolar circle may be adjusted if necessary to accommodate the areola in its new position, keeping the upper pole constant. Lista *et al.*, in their study of vertical reduction mammaplasty,[6] discuss how pedicle choice is dependent on the markings. After the markings are made, if any part of the areola falls within the mosque pattern, a superior dermo-glandular pedicle is used. If the areola is below the mosque pattern, a medial pedicle is used. This facilitates insetting the areola in its new location after the reduction procedure. In oncoplastic procedures, the type of nipple areola pedicle is dictated by the location of the tumor.

In June 2006, Fahmy *et al.* reported from United Kingdom[7] on another technique that makes freehand marking easier, even for surgeons with limited experience. The markings are made with the patient in sitting, supine, and oblique positions. After marking the fixed point of the supra-sternal notch, the breast (nipple) meridian is marked from the clavicle equidistant from the supra-sternal notch on either side and through the center of the nipple, carrying it across the inframammary fold. The new nipple position is marked along the breast meridian. With the patient in the supine position, the inframammary folds are marked with gentle pressure on the breasts and with a dart along the intersection of the breast meridian with the inframammary fold. This avoids tension on wound closure. The medial limb of the vertical ellipse is marked by connecting the new nipple point to the dart in a straight line.

With the patient in an oblique sitting position, as the breasts fall laterally, the lateral limbs of the vertical ellipse are marked, connecting the new nipple point to the inframammary dart in a straight line, marking the right breast with the patient in the left lateral oblique position, and vice versa. Finally, with the patient in an upright sitting position, 7 cm-long medial and lateral limbs are marked from the new nipple point to intersect with the medial and lateral limbs of the vertical ellipse for an inverted "T" reduction. For a vertical scar reduction, new nipple markings are made lower along the breast meridian, and the vertical ellipse is marked with the lower end of the ellipse, ending 2–4 cm above the inframammary fold according to the size of the breast reduction.

## References

1. Penn J. (1955) Breast reduction. *Br J Plast Surg* 7(4):357–371.
2. Westreich M. (1997) Anthropomorphic breast measurement: Protocol and results in 50 women with aesthetically perfect breasts and clinical application. *Plast Reconstr Surg* 100(2):468–479.

3. Smith DJ, Jr., Palin WE, Jr., Katch VL, Bennett JE.(1986) Breast volume and anthropomorphic measurements: Normal values. *Plast Reconstr Surg* 78(3):331–335.
4. Hall-Findlay EJ. (2010) The three breast dimensions: Analysis and effecting change. *Plast Reconstr Surg* 125(6):1632–1642.
5. Bostwick J. (1983) *Aesthetic and Reconstructive Breast Surgery.* The C. V. Mosby Company, St. Louis, Missouri.
6. Lista F, Ahmad J. (2006) Vertical scar reduction mammaplasty: A 15-year experience including a review of 250 consecutive cases. *Plast Reconstr Surg* 117(7):2152–2165; discussion 66–69.
7. Fahmy FS, Hemington-Gorse SJ. (2006) The sitting, oblique, and supine marking technique for reduction mammaplasty and mastopexy. *Plast Reconstr Surg* 17(7):2145–2151.

# Chapter 3

# NEOADJUVANT THERAPY

Laurie Kirstein*, Susan K. Boolbol*, and Mahmoud El-Tamer†

*Division of Breast Surgery,
Beth Israel Medical Center,
New York, NY 10003, USA

†Breast Service, Department of Surgery,
Memorial Sloan-Kettering Cancer Center,
New York, NY 10065, USA

## 3.1 Introduction

Since the publication of large clinical trials showing equivalent survival between mastectomy and lumpectomy followed by radiation for early-stage breast cancer, more women have chosen breast-conserving surgery (BCS).[1] Until recently, however, for patients with more locally advanced tumors or those with a larger tumor-to-breast ratio, mastectomy has remained the mainstay of surgical treatment. In order to achieve the desired cosmetic outcome, these patients with larger tumors were better served with a mastectomy, followed by immediate breast reconstruction.

In the mid-1980s, a new concept emerged that changed the course of treatment for patients with locally advanced breast cancer. A proposal was introduced whereby chemotherapy would be delivered prior to surgery with the goal of decreasing the tumor burden. If successful, the chance of undergoing BCS would be increased.[2] Since then, multiple studies have been undertaken to evaluate the safety and effectiveness of neoadjuvant chemotherapy (NCT) on surgical outcome, overall survival (OS), and disease-free survival (DFS). A pathologic complete response (pCR) is the ultimate goal, as well as a complete clinical response (cCR). Not only does this have the best prognostic significance for the patient, but a cCR also allows for breast conservation in a setting that was not formerly thought possible. In this chapter, the clinical and pathologic response to NCT will be discussed with respect to various breast cancer subtypes. Finally, even patients with partial responses may be eligible for BCS, taking into account techniques to localize tumors, reduce re-excision rates, and increase surgical resection volume, by utilizing oncoplastic reconstructive techniques.

## 3.2 Background

### 3.2.1 *Early Trials*

Neoadjuvant therapy has been in use by surgeons for more than 30 years. The concept of medical therapy prior to surgical resection was first used in patients who were deemed inoperable due to their extent of disease.[3] The first reports were encouraging as the vast majority of patients demonstrated a significant response that was complete by 10% to 15%. This concept was later applied in patients with locally advanced disease with a significant improvement in survival when compared to historical control. In an attempt to study the impact of preoperative chemotherapy on survival, multiple prospective longitudinal and randomized trials were designed.

The National Surgical Adjuvant Breast and Bowel Project (NSABP) B-18 trial evaluated 4 rounds of cyclophosphamide and doxorubicin given either before or after definitive surgery.[4] The results of this landmark trial demonstrated that there was no difference in OS, DFS, or progression-free survival (PFS) regardless of the timing of chemotherapy. In addition, pathologic tumor response correlated to OS, PFS, and DFS. Those patients with a pCR displayed the highest OS, DFS, and PFS. The main difference between the groups was the change in surgical treatment of patients in the NCT group from mastectomy to BCS. In the group of patients who received NCT, there was a significant increase in the number of patients who underwent breast conservation compared to the adjuvant group ($p = 0.001$).[4]

The NSBAP B-27 trial also evaluated NCT with a different regimen than the B-18 trial. The patients were given four rounds of Adriamycin and cytoxan (AC) preoperatively or postoperatively with or without a taxane. Again, although there was no statistically significant difference in OS, DFS, and PFS between the 2 groups, in the neoadjuvant group, BCS was achieved 68% of the time compared with 60% of patients the adjuvant group. The addition of a taxane to the neoadjuvant protocol did not affect the breast conservation rate. About 63% of the patients underwent breast conservation with the addition of the taxane, whereas about 60% used $AC$ alone ($p = NS$).[5]

With these encouraging data to support the option of chemotherapy before surgery, especially in patients who desired breast conservation, additional trials emerged examining the role for this treatment in different groups of breast cancer patients. In 2005, Mieog *et al.* reviewed the Cochrane database and identified 14 randomized controlled trials that they deemed appropriate. These studies compared neoadjuvant with adjuvant chemotherapy in 5,500 women with operable breast cancer (T1–3 N0–2 M0). They reported that NCT downstaged 25.6% of the patients and significantly decreased the mastectomy rate by 16.6% ($p < 0.001$). Only 4.3% of the patients were upstaged.[6]

### 3.2.2 *Patient Selection*

#### 3.2.2.1 *Exclusionary criteria*

There are subsets of patients for whom BCS is contraindicated. These patients may be candidates for NCT for reasons other than breast conservation. A patient with 2 or more cancers in different quadrants, or multicentric disease, would not be a candidate for breast conservation but may still undergo NCT. In the ideal situation, in which this patient achieves a cCR, she would not be a candidate for breast conservation. In general, it is unusual to perform multiple lumpectomies in different quadrants. We continue to recommend excision of the tumor bed after NCT even in patients who have achieved a complete clinical and radiological response. We believe at this time that the only objective evidence of response remains the pathologic evaluation of the tumor site. Furthermore, all patients receiving NCT are advised to receive postoperative radiation therapy to the whole breast with a boost dose to the tumor bed. While cosmesis is important, it is the penultimate consideration, with oncologic principles being the most important.

Although currently, the standard of care in inflammatory carcinoma is NCT, we have avoided BCS in these patients. The risk of local recurrence is significantly high; hence, we feel that mastectomy after NCT remains the optimal surgical procedure. Extensive microcalcifications that are beyond the realm of breast conservation are another contraindication to NCT for the aim of BCS. It has been our experience that although tumor masses respond well to NCT with partial or complete radiologic response, microcalcifications tend to persist and have to be totally excised during any attempt at BCS to confirm pathologic response. Other relative contraindications are patients with extensive cutaneous involvement where resection would necessitate tissue coverage. In these clinical scenarios, we have recommended primary surgery with a mastectomy.

### 3.2.3 *Tumor Size*

Historically, tumors larger than 4 cm to 5 cm were considered too large for BCS, and mastectomy was recommended. Therefore, this was the initial group of patients considered eligible for NCT.[7] The goal in this situation was to decrease the size of the tumor and thereby render the patient eligible for breast conservation.[8] The early trials revealed a significant increase in breast conservation compared to mastectomy for this very group of patients, ranging from 23% to 32%.[5]

The current National Cancer Center Network (NCCN) guidelines recommend consideration of NCT for patients with clinical stage IIa cancer (T2 N0 M0).[9] One must remember that size alone does not dictate the need for NCT. The tumor-to-breast size ratio and the location of the cancer are points that need to be evaluated when considering surgical options. For example, even a 2 cm-diameter tumor in a woman with small A-cup breasts may not result in an acceptable cosmetic result with BCS. Should the patient need adjuvant therapy for this tumor, consideration should be given to NCT in order to decrease the size of the tumor and provide a better cosmetic outcome (see Case No. 1).

Case No. 1

The patient was 49 years old with a palpable mass in the right breast that was clinically 2 cm in size. Ultrasound and mammogram have revealed a highly suspicious lesion in the lower outer quadrant of the right breast corresponding to the palpable area of concern. On ultrasound interrogation, the mass measured 1.8 cm × 1.5 cm × 2.3 cm. A core needle biopsy confirmed the diagnosis of an invasive ductal carcinoma (estrogen/progesterone receptor negative HER2neu 3+). Two abnormal nodes were confirmed to harbor metastatic disease by needle biopsy. The patient was interested in BCS. Her breast cup size was A-AA. She received NCT, AC, and T with herceptin. She underwent a lumpectomy and axillary node dissection. The pathology revealed 0.3 cm residual disease in the breast and that all 24 axillary nodes were free of metastasis.

(a–b) The patient 6 months after completion of radiation therapy.

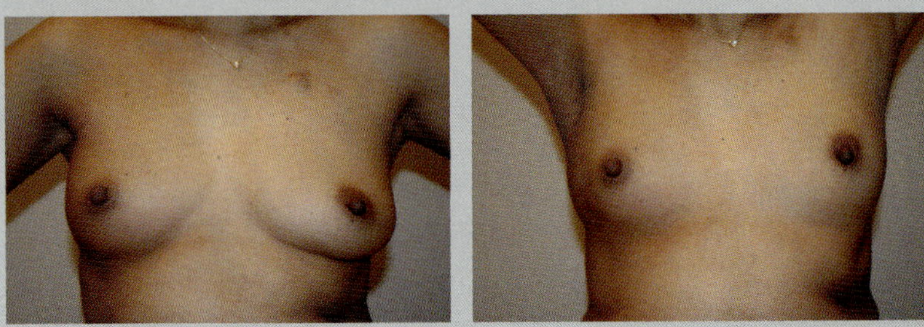

(a) (b)

Image 1.1

## 3.3 Staging

### 3.3.1 *Current Staging Guidelines*

Patients who are candidates for NCT are those with larger tumors or with clinically palpable lymph nodes; therefore it is important to rule out metastatic disease prior to initiation of treatment. The current NCCN guidelines recommend a metastatic workup for patients with stage IIb cancers or higher, similar to the group of patients who would be considered for NCT.[9] NCCN staging guidelines consist of blood work, a chest X-ray, a computerized axial tomography (CAT) scan of the abdomen and pelvis, and a bone scan. Any abnormalities should be further evaluated with subsequent imaging or a positron emission tomography/CAT scan. For example, an abnormality on a bone scan may lead to magnetic resonance imaging (MRI) of the suspicious lesion or an 18F-fluorodeoxyglucose-positron emission tomography (FDG-PET) scan to assess the lesion for metabolic activity. It is also important to obtain pathologic confirmation of metastatic disease because this will render the patient stage IV and alter the treatment plan.

### 3.3.2 *The Role of Imaging*

The ultimate goal of NCT is to eradicate the tumor. Often this means the tumor's appearance after chemotherapy is drastically different compared with its appearance prior to initiation of treatment, both radiographically and clinically. This highlights the importance of thoroughly evaluating malignant lesions with imaging studies not only prior to the initiation of chemotherapy but also prior to surgical treatment. This also reinforces the need to place a tumor marker prior to the initiation of chemotherapy.[10] There are instances in which the patient has a complete radiologic response and the tumor marker is needed in order to proceed with breast conservation with needle localization.

### 3.3.3 *Mammogram*

The importance of assessing the extent of the tumor prior to NCT is paramount. Often this workup begins with a clinical breast examination and standard imaging modalities, consisting of mammography and sonography. Mammography is usually the initial imaging modality used to evaluate the breast, either before or after diagnosis of carcinoma. While mammography has been shown to be more accurate in patients with less-dense parenchyma, it can also be helpful in detecting calcifications in or surrounding a lesion. However, mammograms are more limited when evaluating tumors located in the far posterior breast against the chest wall.[11]

Mammography also incompletely visualizes nodal basins other than the low axilla. In 2 small studies, mammography alone or in combination with clinical breast exam detected invasive breast cancers in about 81% to 86% of patients with known disease.[12,13] As an adjunct to mammography, the ultrasound examination of the breast can be useful in the context of a more complete assessment of the breast prior to treatment.[12]

It has been our observation that microcalcifications do not resolve with NCT in spite of good pathologic response. All suspicious residual microcalcifications seen around the tumor bed should be completely excised during surgical intervention. Hence patients who present with extensive microcalcifications that cannot be excised by breast conservation and an oncoplastic procedure should have a mastectomy.

### 3.3.4 *Ultrasonography*

In the early neoadjuvant trials, a physical exam with calipers and ultrasound measurement of the tumor was standard. In the same trials already listed, diagnostic ultrasonography detected 94% to 97% of invasive breast cancers, and detected multifocal or multicentric disease in a total of 14% of patients.[12,13] For patients who are being evaluated for breast conservation, it is important to obtain tissue diagnosis of all suspected lesions prior to initiation of NCT. This will allow for an evaluation after chemotherapy to assess treatment response, as well as direct surgical planning. It may also exclude patients with multicentric disease for breast conservation.

Mammography and sonography may be used to not only perform a percutaneous needle biopsy to confirm the presence of the tumor but also to leave a metal-marking clip in the area of biopsy.[10] Some physicians prefer to leave a clip at the center of the tumor, while others prefer to mark the areas of tumor which are furthest apart, which may have implications for the volume of surgical resection needed. We have relied on a clip in the center of the tumor as we limit our resection to the residual disease, and we do not necessarily excise all of the original tumor bed if the patient had achieved a pathologic response to chemotherapy. Confirmation of proper clip placement should be obtained with a postplacement mammogram, even if the clip is placed by ultrasound guidance. Again, these markers are of the utmost importance in the case of a complete radiologic response. In this situation, the clips are the only evidence of the location of the prior tumor. If breast conservation is performed, these clips can then be used for needle localization at the time of definitive surgery. In patients with multiple lesions, differently shaped metallic clips should be placed in each lesion to help direct which area to excise after completion of chemotherapy if breast conservation becomes an option.

Ultrasonography can be helpful not only in measurement of primary breast tumors but also in assessment of nodal basins. The appearance of a lymph node with a change in architecture consisting of a thickened cortex or loss of the fatty hilum leads to the suspicion of regional metastatic disease. These characteristics of macrometastatic disease are easily seen by utilizing current ultrasound technology. Ultrasonography has difficulty visualizing micrometastases, and therefore pathologic evaluation is still necessary.[11,14] Krishnamurthy *et al.* reported results comparing ultrasound-guided fine needle aspiration (FNA) of suspicious axillary lymph nodes with those excised at complete axillary node dissection.[14] FNA correctly identified positive lymph nodes in all patients who had 3 or more positive lymph nodes. It also correctly identified positive lymph nodes in 93% of patients who had a metastatic deposit $>0.5$ mm. The sensitivity of the ultrasound-guided FNA of the axillary lymph node was 86%, and the specificity was 100%. The positive predictive value was 100%, and the negative predictive value was 67%, with an overall diagnostic accuracy of 79%. Ultrasonography can be used to evaluate not only the axillary lymph nodes but also the internal mammary and supraclavicular nodes.

Although not performed routinely, targeted ultrasonography can be used as an adjunct to an abnormal clinical finding or a radiologic abnormality after NCT. A change in the appearance of lymph nodes after chemotherapy might indicate a response to treatment and can be valuable prognostically.[15] The information obtained from an axillary ultrasound can be invaluable. This aside, pathologic evaluation of the lymph node needs to be performed during treatment, whether it is prior to or after NCT, for ultimate surgical and radiation treatment planning.

### 3.3.5 *Magnetic Resonance Imaging (MRI)*

Functional imaging has emerged as a helpful tool in the assessment of breast cancer patients eligible for NCT. For newly diagnosed breast cancer patients, MRI has a sensitivity $>90\%$.[16] However, more importantly, up to 10% of patients with a newly diagnosed breast cancer have an occult lesion detected by MRI in either the ipsilateral or contralateral breast.[16] Finally, MRI is superior to mammography at visualizing far posterior lesions, including those with chest-wall involvement.[11]

In patients being considered for NCT, it is important to biopsy any suspicious lesions detected by MRI. Biopsy can be performed via MRI if necessary, but also by targeted ultrasonography or mammography if the lesion is seen on these studies subsequent to the diagnostic MRI. This allows for adequate stratification of patients who remain eligible for NCT and identifies lesions that need to be excised at definitive surgery. It is important to remember to leave a clip in any area where an image-guided biopsy is performed.[10]

Some studies have shown that MRI is more accurate at predicting residual disease after NCT than mammography or ultrasonography.[17,18] In fact, it has been suggested that a pCR can be predicted by lack of residual enhancement on a postneoadjuvant MRI. This is an advantage of functional imaging in that an MRI not only measures the static size of the tumor but also the viability of the tumor cells by using contrast-enhancing kinetics.[19] For example, after NCT, some masses are still present on physical exam and standard imaging. On MRI, however, some of these tumors no longer take up gadolinium in a suspicious pattern, indicating these cells are likely necrotic from the chemotherapy. Rather than relying on a clinical exam in which a palpable mass is still present after NCT, an MRI, revealing a decrease in suspicious uptake, may more confidently allow for a recommendation for an attempt at breast conservation and decrease the surgical resection volume. Performing an MRI prior to and after NCT can be a helpful adjunct to assess tumor response and has become an integral part of the workup of the patient undergoing NCT.[20] It has been our personal experience, however, that lack of uptake of gadolinium may be related to partial disruption of vascular supply of the tumor without complete pathologic response.

One of the most important aspects with respect to imaging in the neoadjuvant patient is to repeat the studies after treatment. Using a combination of modalities — mammography, ultrasonography, MRI, and clinical examination — increases the sensitivity and more accurately measures residual tumor size. This allows for both assessment of tumor response and better surgical planning.[11] The surgeon has to be cognizant that if MRI is used as the sole measure of tumor size, this may lead to more extensive surgery. Houssami *et al.* reported MRI led to more extensive surgery in 11% of cases and resulted in unnecessary conversion to mastectomy in between 3% and 33% of cases (average: 8%).[21]

## 3.4 Predictors of Response

It is helpful to know which patients will have an appropriate response to chemotherapy in order to help stratify those patients who will be eligible for breast conservation. This allows the surgeon and the medical oncologist to set appropriate expectations. In addition, it allows for planning of chemotherapy regimens according to tumor biology. Overall, there is a wide range in the response to NCT. The measurements of response include both clinical and pathologic response. In general, patients with triple negative and HER2 positive biologic profiles have a higher overall response rate, both clinically and pathologically. Tumors that are hormone receptor-positive have lower clinical and pathologic response rates.

NCT may cause cancer cells to respond in numerous ways that affect the subsequent size and shape of the residual tumor. Some tumors have a response in the majority of the cells that causes them to shrink in a concentric pattern. These tumors exhibit a decrease in their overall size, possibly making them eligible for breast conservation after treatment. This is in contrast to other tumors that do not achieve the same reliable pattern of response. These tumors may have a heterogeneous response to treatment, which leaves islands of treated cells intermingled with viable cancer cells. Unfortunately, these tumors still retain most of their original overall size and may contribute to the failure of breast conservation in this population. Examining the different biological subtypes of breast cancer sheds light on the response to treatment and the likelihood of achieving breast conservation.

### 3.4.1 *Response to NCT Based on Molecular Subtype*

#### 3.4.1.1 *Triple negative*

Approximately 15% of all breast cancers are estrogen and progesterone receptor negative and HER2 receptor negative, otherwise known as triple-negative breast cancer (TNBC). As a group, these tumors tend to be more aggressive with poorer outcomes. One of the traditional choices of chemotherapy for TNBC has included anthracycline-based regimes and taxanes. Recent studies have also examined the role of platinum-based chemotherapy in the patient with TNBC. There are also a number of emerging targets in this particular population, including the poly-ADP-ribose-polymerase (PARP) inhibitors, which have recently been included in select neoadjuvant trials. It appears from numerous studies that patients with TNBC have the highest clinical and pathologic response to NCT. This fact increases the number of patients potentially eligible for breast conservation after NCT.

In the largest series published to date, Liedtke *et al.* described the pCR rate in their series of 225 TNBC patients who received NCT. This group was compared to 863 patients not having TNBC who also underwent NCT. In this study, 22% of the TNBC patients achieved a pCR compared with 11% in non-TNBC patients ($p = 0.034$).[22] This is in keeping with previously reported numbers in smaller studies in which the range of pCR ranged from 27% to 38%.[23,24] The authors of this study noted an increased pCR rate in patients treated solely with different anthracycline-based regimens with or without a prior taxane. In this study by Liedtke *et al.*, there was not a significant pCR for a single agent-based taxane regimen, but only a trend.

In addition to tumor response, this study also reported final surgical treatment in the TNBC versus non-TNBC groups. Those patients with TNBC and a pCR, or 22% of the group, should have been eligible for BCS after NCT. Encouragingly, this number was higher than 22%, with 40% of TNBC patients undergoing BCS compared with 30% of non-TNBC patients. This would indicate that even patients with only partial responses were able to achieve breast conservation, perhaps with larger surgical volume.

Platinum-based chemotherapy regimens are another group of agents that have been investigated in the setting of TNBCs. Platinum-based therapies have been utilized in this population as second-line treatment or for metastatic disease for some time, but only recently have they been utilized for a few small neoadjuvant trials. In one such trial, 22 patients with TNBC were treated with cisplatin monotherapy, and 5 (23%) of the patients had a pCR.[25] In another small study, a group of BRCA-1 mutation carriers with TNBC achieved a 72% pCR.[26] However, the surgical outcome was not reported, but theoretically, all of these patients would be eligible for BCS. Given this information, platinum-based agents may hold promise in some patients with TNBC and allow them to achieve breast conservation. A list of pCR rates based on different chemotherapy regimens for TNBC can be found in Table 3.1.

#### 3.4.1.2 *HER2 positive*

Another group of locally advanced breast cancer (LABC) patients in whom NCT holds promise for BCS are those with HER2 positive tumors.

Table 3.1. Pathologic complete response rates in triple-negative breast cancer (TNBC) patients in the neoadjuvant setting.[62]

| Study | Chemotherapy regimen | pCR rate |
|---|---|---|
| Dana Farber | Cisplatin | 22% |
| MGH/Dana Farber/BID | Cisplatin +/− bevacizumab | 16% |
| Pomeranian Medical University (BRCA1 + patients) | Cisplatin | 72% |
| University of Texas MD Anderson Cancer Center | Retrospective various regimens | 22% |
| University of Texas MD Anderson Cancer Center | Retrospective paclitaxel followed by FAC[a] | 45% |

[a]5-fluorouracil, doxorubicin, cyclophosphamide (FAC). pCR, pathologic complete response.

Table 3.2. Pathologic clinical response to neoadjuvant chemotherapy with or without trastuzumab for HER2 overexpressing tumors.

| Study | With trastuzumab | Without trastuzumab |
|---|---|---|
| Buzdar[27] | 65% | 26% |
| Paluch-Shimon[29] | 75% | 24% |
| Peintinger[30] | 73% | 34% |

Multiple randomized trials have now been published, demonstrating a higher rate of pCR rates to NCT with the addition of trastuzumab for HER2-overexpressing tumors (Table 3.2).[27–30]

In 2005, data from Buzdar *et al.*[27] demonstrated a 62.5% pCR rate with the addition of trastuzumab to a neoadjuvant protocol of four cycles of paclitaxel plus fluorouracil (5FU), epirubicin, and cyclophosphamide (FEC), compared to a 26% pCR with conventional chemotherapy in the neoadjuvant setting, without increase in clinical congestive heart failure. This was irrespective of hormone status, although patients with hormone-positive tumors received endocrine treatment for 5 years in the adjuvant setting. Although the trial was small and only enrolled 34 patients, it was closed early due to the superiority of the trastuzumab arm. Subsequent trials, both prospective and retrospective, have demonstrated similar findings.[27]

This same group then published data in which they examined the effect of hormone-receptor status on the pCR rate.[30] The trial included the potential addition of trastuzumab with various combinations of standard NCT. There were multiple variables, including dosing schedules of taxol weekly or once every 3 weeks, followed by 5-fluorouracil, doxorubicin or epirubicin, and cyclophosphamide. The results demonstrated that patients with hormone receptor positive-tumors had a significantly higher pCR with the addition of trastuzumab. The highest pCR rate of 73% was achieved in the group receiving trastuzumab plus 3-weekly taxol followed by FEC. These findings were similar to the pCR rate seen in hormone receptor-negative patients who also received trastuzumab with the neoadjuvant protocol.[30]

Early in 2010, the results from the neoadjuvant herceptin (NOAH) trial were released in which patients with locally advanced or inflammatory breast cancer were given either NCT with trastuzumab followed by adjuvant trastuzumab, or chemotherapy alone.[28] This trial also included an HER2 negative cohort treated with the same chemotherapy regimen, which consisted of doxorubicin, paclitaxel, cyclophosphamide, methotrexate, and 5-fluoruracil. Results of this trial demonstrated improved event-free survival, OS, and clinical and pathologic tumor responses.

Remembering that a pCR leads to a higher rate of breast conservation, the addition of trastuzumab to NCT regimens for patients with HER2 positive tumors naturally suggests a higher rate of BCS in this group of patients.

### 3.5 Gene Profiling

Some researchers have evaluated the role of the 70-gene profile (Mammaprint®) in predicting response. Straver *et al.*[31] categorized the tumors of 167 patients by using the 70-gene profile and identified 23 patients with good prognosis signature and 144 with poor prognosis signature or poor prognosis. All patients had received NCT. None of the good signature prognosis patients achieved a pCR in the breast and axilla, whereas 20% in the poor prognosis group had no residual tumor identified in the breast and axilla ($p = 0.015$). When looking for pCR or near pCR in the breast, only 2 of 14 (9%) in the good prognosis group compared to 53 of 144 (37%) in the poor prognosis group ($p = 0.008$) achieved that end point.

### 3.6 Hormone Receptor-Positive Tumors

Multiple studies have demonstrated a reduced pCR to NCT for hormone receptor-positive tumors.[32] With this observation, the question became whether a better method existed to reduce the size of locally advanced breast cancers in the hormone receptor-positive population to facilitate breast conservation. This led to the undertaking of trials that examined the effect of neoadjuvant hormonal therapy with either tamoxifen or an aromatase inhibitor (AI) on these tumors. While trials examining the effect of NCT in the TNBC and HER2 positive breast cancer patient tend to report clinical and pathologic response rates, which can be used as a surrogate for potential for BCS, pCR rates for tumors treated with neoadjuvant hormonal therapy tend to be low, in the order of approximately 2% to 3%.[32] Rather, these trials report clinical response rates and percentage of patients undergoing BCS, which is much more in keeping with the focus of this chapter (Table 3.3).[4,33,34]

For premenopausal women, the choice for neoadjuvant hormonal therapy is tamoxifen or ovarian suppression with an AI, much like adjuvant treatment. However, there is little data available for neoadjuvant tamoxifen in the premenopausal patient. This is because premenopausal women with LABC are more likely to be offered chemotherapy in a neoadjuvant setting rather than hormonal treatment. The postmenopausal patient with

Table 3.3. Pathologic clinical response rate to neoadjuvant chemotherapy, based on tumor hormone status.

| Study | Estrogen receptor-positive | Estrogen receptor-negative |
|---|---|---|
| Buzdar, 2003[33] | 5% | 21% |
| Tan, 2009[34] | 10% | 54% |
| Rastogi, 2008[4] | 6% | 14% |

breast cancer has been more rigorously studied in the neoadjuvant hormonal setting. In this population, the reported breast conservation rate for neoadjuvant tamoxifen is in the range of 30% to 35%.[35,36] However, since aromatase inhibitors are the first line of treatment for postmenopausal women with hormone receptor-positive breast cancer, the main focus of research has been on this group of medications.

The results from the first clinical trial comparing tamoxifen to an AI, anastrozole or tamoxifen alone, or in a combination (ATAC) trial, showed that anastrozole was superior to tamoxifen alone or with both drugs in combination with respect to DFS in the adjuvant setting.[37] Based on these findings, the immediate preoperative anastrozole, tamoxifen, or combined with tamoxifen (IMPACT) trial, a multicenter, double-blind randomized trial that compared anastrozole alone, tamoxifen alone, or both drugs in combination, was developed in the neoadjuvant setting.[36] Patients were given the determined medication for 12 weeks prior to surgery. The primary endpoint was clinical overall response rate. Although, there was no statistically significant difference in overall response between patients treated with anastrozole or tamoxifen alone, there was a trend. In subgroup analyses of patients who were deemed to need a mastectomy prior to treatment, there was a significantly different number of patients who were downgraded from mastectomy to breast conservation in both medication groups (44% versus 22%, $p = 0.03$). However, when subset analyses examined the surgical outcome in each medication group, 45% of patients initially requiring mastectomy were downgraded to breast conservation after neoadjuvant anastrozole compared to 36% of patients after tamoxifen. This trial concluded that neoadjuvant anastrozole was more effective at downstaging patients than tamoxifen.

Similarly, the preoperative arimidex compared to tamoxifen (PROACT) trial sought to compare each single agent with or without chemotherapy in the neoadjuvant setting with respect to overall response measured by clinical exam and ultrasonography, as well as rate of downgrading to breast conservation.[38] This large, randomized, double-blind, double-dummy trial found that anastrozole was at least as effective as tamoxifen in obtaining an overall response and breast conservation rate, but not statistically different. Together, the results of the IMPACT and PROACT trials showed that anastrozole was as effective or better then tamoxifen as a single agent in the neoadjuvant setting in postmenopausal women at achieving a clinical response and downstaging to BCS.[36,38]

The use of neoadjuvant letrozole was studied in the P024 trial, another large, multinational, double-blind trial in which letrozole alone versus tamoxifen alone was given for 4 months prior to surgery in hormone receptor-positive patients who were not eligible for BCS.[32] The primary endpoints were clinical and pathologic response rate determined by clinical breast exam, with the secondary endpoint being the percentage of patients who underwent BCS. The overall response to letrozole was found to be statistically significantly higher than to tamoxifen (55% versus 36%, $p < 0.001$). In addition, significantly more patients receiving neoadjuvant letrozole were able to achieve breast conservation compared with those taking tamoxifen (45% versus 35%, $p = 0.02$). Interestingly, in this study, patients who were HER2 positive were found to have a higher overall response rate with letrozole compared to tamoxifen ($p = 0.0004$). The overall response rate for patients with HER2 positive, estrogen-receptor positive breast cancers taking letrozole was similar to that of patients with HER2 negative tumors (71%). Letrozole was also found to be more effective than tamoxifen in tumors that were marginally estrogen-receptor positive. The conclusion from the P024 trial was that letrozole was more effective than tamoxifen at inducing an overall response to treatment and downgrading patients requiring mastectomy to BCS. Further studies have confirmed these findings.[32]

The final aromatase inhibitor, examestane, has been examined in the neoadjuvant setting in smaller, phase II trials. Of the 221 total patients in these trials, the overall response rate ranged from 34% to 73%, with 56% to 76% of patients undergoing BCS (Table 3.4).[32,36,39–42]

Table 3.4. Percentage of breast-conserving surgery (BCS) with neoadjuvant hormonal therapy.

| Hormone treatment | Study | BCS, % |
|---|---|---|
| Tamoxifen | IMPACT[36] | 36 |
| | P024[32] | 35 |
| Anastrozole | IMPACT[36] | 44 |
| Letrozole | P024[32] | 45 |
| Examestane | Barnadas[39] | 56 |
| | Mlineritsch[40] | 76 |
| | Takei[41] | 90 |
| | Tubiana-Hulin[42] | 57 |

Now that it has been shown that aromatase inhibitors are effective at achieving a good clinical response with possible downstaging from mastectomy to breast conservation, it is important to ascertain which patients are likely to benefit from hormone therapy alone rather than in combination with chemotherapy. In the adjuvant setting, there are genomic assays that stratify patients into groups according to recurrence risk. Those tumors with low recurrence risk do not benefit from the addition of chemotherapy to hormonal treatment. Conversely, in those patients with tumors with a high risk of recurrence, the addition of chemotherapy confers a benefit to endocrine treatment (OncotypeDX®, MammaPrint®). It may be helpful to use this information in a neoadjuvant setting to determine if a patient will benefit from the addition of NCT in addition to neoadjuvant hormones.

One study in the literature examined whether a 21-gene assay could predict response to neoadjuvant treatment with tamoxifen or anastrozole.[43] The recurrence scores were based upon pretreatment core biopsies. Only half of the samples yielded enough RNA for examination. The results showed that patients with low recurrence scores tended to have a better response to neoadjuvant hormonal therapy than those with intermediate or high recurrence scores, regardless of which hormonal therapy was used. This was a small pilot study, but opens an interesting new area of study with respect to tumor genomics and individualized neoadjuvant treatment.

## 3.7 Invasive Lobular Carcinoma

Patients with lobular carcinoma tend not to have as favorable a response to NCT as those with ductal carcinoma.[44] Perhaps it is the morphologic features of lobular carcinoma and its tendency to have multiple islands of tumor over distances which confer a poor response. It may also be attributed to the fact that the vast majority of lobular tumors are strongly hormone receptor-positive and HER2 receptor-negative. As previously stated, the response of hormone receptor-positive tumors to NCT is not as good as their estrogen receptor-negative counterparts. Therefore, for a patient with invasive lobular carcinoma, one must adequately rule out multicentricity and one should consider neoadjuvant hormonal therapy if breast conservation is desired.[45]

## 3.8 Surgery After NCT

### 3.8.1 *Surgical Decision Making*

There are still a fair number of patients who undergo mastectomy after NCT who on pathologic review are found to have a pCR. For example,

Buzdar reported a 50% breast conservation rate after NCT in a group of patients in whom there was a 65% pCR rate.[27] This lends itself to the question of what factors contribute to surgical recommendations. The major factors that lead to a final surgical decision seem to include persistence of a mass on clinical exam, persistence of imaging abnormality, and patient preference.[5,46]

Considering that patient preference for unilateral or bilateral mastectomy is a factor that is not necessarily under a physician's control, the other contributing factors — presence of a mass or imaging abnormality — should be addressed prior to surgical recommendation. Although the presence of a mass may indicate residual tumor cells, it may not represent viable disease. As noted in the previous imaging section, mammography or sonography may show residual mass or density, but MRI may not reveal suspicious enhancement kinetics. After NCT, it is important to adequately assess the amount of viable tumor before making surgical recommendations; an MRI is a valuable tool in this process.

### 3.8.2 *Resection Volume and Margins*

As with any other breast-conservation procedure, it is just as important to obtain clear margins when performing surgery after NCT. It is well known that tumor cells at the inked edge of a specimen carry a high risk of local recurrence. Since there are variable response patterns to tumors undergoing NCT, careful evaluation of specimen margins is paramount. It is also important to take into account the pattern of response histopathologically, and correlate this with preoperative imaging. Should a tumor have a heterogeneous response, it is theoretically possible to dissect between islands of tumor to have a seemingly clear margin. It behooves the surgeon and pathologist to review and report the pattern of tumor response to treatment and then compare the tissue to preoperative MRI. Should there be any doubt as to the response pattern, or if there was questionable enhancement on MRI prior to surgery, either the MRI should be repeated or re-excision should be performed.

The important concept to remember when operating on a patient after NCT is that one is removing only the tumor that is present after chemotherapy and not what was once there before the initiation of treatment. This means that resection volume should be smaller after NCT. This is why it is important to mark the center of a tumor with a metal marker clip prior to initiation of treatment rather than the areas of the tumor that are farthest apart.[10] Should a surgeon remove the entire area between edges of the previous viable tumor, this negates the effect of NCT. Theoretically, if the furthest edges of the mass have been marked prior to chemotherapy, as the mass regresses, the clips should move closer together. This also facilitates a smaller resection volume.

For patients who do not achieve a pCR, breast conservation may still be attempted. Studies have shown that using multiple localizing wires may help achieve breast conservation for larger lesions with fewer re-excisions.[47] In one such study, 77.1% of patients with larger breast cancer had successful BCS by utilizing multiple localizing wires, with 28% requiring more than one excision to achieve clear margins.[48] Utilizing oncoplastic techniques in larger volume resections can help maintain cosmesis in these cases with larger resection volumes.

Finally, it is important to remove any residual calcifications seen on imaging after completion of chemotherapy. This is because calcifications may represent intraductal disease, which does not respond to chemotherapy. A mammogram prior to surgery can aid in surgical planning for patients with residual calcifications. Ultimately, the decision for breast conservation, and the decision on the number of operations that should be performed to attempt this, belongs in a discussion between patient and surgeon, and plays a role in the individualized care of each breast cancer patient.[5]

### 3.8.3 *Axillary Evaluation*

In the surgical literature, the timing of axillary evaluation in the patient receiving NCT is a current controversy. There are multiple studies supporting axillary evaluation prior to chemotherapy as well as afterward.

### 3.8.4 *Sentinel Node Biopsy Prior to NCT*

It is accepted that the false-negative rate of sentinel node biopsy is $< 5\%$. Early studies which evaluated the sentinel lymph node after chemotherapy reported false-negative rates of up to 10%, which some clinicians felt was unacceptably high.[49] In addition, radiation planning may be affected by the timing of the sentinel node biopsy. If a sentinel node contains metastatic disease prior to NCT, then a full axillary dissection is performed at the time of definitive surgery, which may or may not lead to the diagnosis of additional metastatic nodes. Conventional radiation planning is based on 4 or more involved lymph nodes. There are some patients, however, who might be offered comprehensive radiation after breast conservation or postmastectomy radiation with only 1 or more involved lymph nodes if other tumor factors are present, such as lymphovascular invasion, extracapsular extension, or high mitotic index. If a metastatic sentinel node is not evaluated prior to NCT and is then sterilized by the chemotherapy, the information regarding that node is lost, and comprehensive or postmastectomy radiation may not be offered. Recent meta-analyses involving patients with just 1 to 3 positive lymph nodes who did not receive postmastectomy radiation had a poorer DFS and OS.[50] In fact, many radiation oncologists prefer to know the status of the lymph nodes prior to NCT in order to optimize the radiation fields.

### 3.8.5 *Sentinel Node Biopsy After NCT*

There are also data to support the performing of a sentinel lymph node biopsy after NCT. The sentinel node detection rate post-NCT has varied from 89% to 97%. The false-negative rate has been reported to vary from 10% to 12%.[49,51,52]

The theoretical concept is the same for the axilla as it is for the breast; why remove tissue that does not contain tumor? Just as a smaller volume of resection in the breast is the norm in most patients undergoing NCT, an axillary lymph node dissection in a patient without lymph node metastases has no therapeutic value and subjects the patient to increased morbidity. If the sentinel node is the only node involved with tumor in approximately 60% of patients, and the sentinel node is sterilized by chemotherapy, then there should be no residual tumor in the axilla in the majority of patients, obviating the need for a completion axillary dissection. Furthermore, NCT has been shown to downstage the axilla in 20.0% to 37.5% of patients.[31,53]

Straver *et al.* identified 3 predictors of cPR in axillary nodes: triple negative tumor; HER2-neu positive tumor; and when there is complete pathologic response in the breast primary. By following the same concept of NCT converting patients from mastectomy to BCT, one can extrapolate that by downstaging the axilla, 20.0% to 37.5% of the patients may be spared an unnecessary axillary node dissection if the sentinel node is performed after completion axillary node dissection.

A recent study published by Hunt *et al.* reported their experience with timing of sentinel node surgery prior to or after NCT. In this large retrospective trial from 1994 to 2007, there was no difference in the sentinel node identification rate.[54] More importantly, there was no difference in local recurrence based on timing of the sentinel node biopsy. Criticisms of this trial include the fact that only 15% of patients underwent sentinel node biopsy after chemotherapy and that there was no reporting of radiation fields, which also contributes to local control. Follow-up was not addressed since this was a retrospective study.

A current trial by the American College of Surgeons Oncology Group is designed to answer the questions of whether a sentinel node biopsy is reliable after chemotherapy and what percentage of the time the axilla is sterilized by NCT. In this trial, patients undergoing NCT who are clinically node negative will undergo axillary ultrasound, with aspiration of any suspicious node prior to initiation of chemotherapy. If positive, the patient then goes on to sentinel node biopsy and completion axillary dissection after completion of NCT. The results from this trial will be eagerly anticipated.

Until further data are available, evaluation of the axilla must be performed for the patient undergoing NCT. This may be done prior to or after chemotherapy, depending on the decision of the multidisciplinary team and the patient.

## 3.9 Locoregional Failure: Incidence and Predictors

There have been multiple series in the literature that have reported series rates of local and regional failure post-NCT in patients who underwent breast conservation (Table 3.5). The rate of local and regional recurrence seems to have decreased over the years; this can be attributed to multiple factors, including improvement in chemotherapy regimens, development of targeted therapies, and perhaps better selection criteria. The 5-year rate of locoregional recurrence (LRR) in the modern series over the past 12 years has been around 8%, and the 10-year rate has been around 12%. Such rates are quite encouraging and seem to be consistent among different centers. Such relatively low recurrence rates are likely related to a selection bias as

Table 3.5. Rates of local and regional failure post-neoadjuvant chemotherapy in patients who underwent breast conservation.

| Trial | Year | Follow-up, mos | % Locoregional recurrence BCS | |
|---|---|---|---|---|
| | | | 5 years | 10 years |
| Institut Bergonie[63] | 1991 | 124 | 23 | |
| Institut Curie[64] | 2001 | 93 | 16 | 21.5 |
| NSABP B-18 | 1998 | 60 | 7.9 | |
| Milan CI[65] | 1998 | 96 | 6.8 (8 years) | |
| University of Texas MD Anderson Cancer Center[66] | 2004 | 60 | 8.5 | |
| University of North Carolina[67] | 2002 | 70 | 10 | |
| Schwartz[68] | 2006 | 75 | 7 | 12 |

BCS, breast-conserving surgery.

patients who undergo breast conservation are those who have achieved a significant response to chemotherapy to permit breast conservation.

## 3.10 Predictors of Relapse

### 3.10.1 *Tumor and Patient Characteristics*

There are many patient and tumor factors that may contribute to relapse after NCT. For example, Liedtke *et al.* reported a significantly decreased PFS, a poorer PFS for patients who presented at a younger age, ductal versus non-ductal histology, high nuclear grade, and high tumor stage.[22] They also noted a decreased PFS for patients with TNBC compared with non-TNBC (63% versus 76%). In fact, presence of the estrogen receptor or progesterone receptor was associated with increased PFS, while the presence of the HER2 receptor showed a trend toward decreased PFS.

A prognostic index was developed and validated by a group at the University of Texas MD Anderson Cancer Center to predict LRR after NCT. The scoring system relies on 4 predictors of ipsilateral and locoregional tumor recurrence: Clinical N2 or N3 disease; residual pathologic tumor size $>2$ cm; a multifocal pattern of residual disease; and lymphovascular invasion. The scoring system assigns a score of 0 (favorable) or 1 (unfavorable) to each criterion based on the presence or absence of each of these factors. The final score is derived by adding the result from each individual variable with 5 possible final categories (0, 1, 2, 3, 4). In patients with scores of 0, 1, or 2, the risk of LRR was the same for those who underwent breast conservation or mastectomy. For patients with scores of 3 or 4, the risk of LRR was significantly higher for those who underwent breast conservation when compared to mastectomy; however, the disease-specific survival was similar. Such scoring may be helpful in selecting patients for breast conservation after NCT.[55,56]

### 3.10.2 *Residual Disease After NCT*

The strongest predictor of relapse after NCT is failure of a pCR.[57,58] It has been shown that patients with residual disease after NCT have decreased DFS and OS. When examining TNBC patients, those patients who do not achieve a pCR have a decrease in OS, whereas TNBC patients who achieve a pCR have a similar OS to non-TNBC patients.[22,24] Similarly, patients with overexpression of the HER2 receptor who did not achieve pCR were found to have a higher likelihood of relapse.[23]

In the TNBC population, it has also been shown that the risk of relapse and death is highest in the first 3 years after treatment. After that time period, the risk of relapse and death is similar to or even lower than non-TNBC patients.[22] Since current NCCN guidelines recommend follow-up staging studies only for symptomatic patients, it becomes important to carefully follow those patients treated with NCT, especially those with residual disease. Surgical treatment of local failure should consist of a mastectomy if the patient still has a breast, or excision of chest wall recurrence, in combination with adjuvant regimens.

## 3.11 Future Directions

### 3.11.1 *PARP Inhibitors*

There are a number of novel therapies in phase II or III trials in the neoadjuvant setting for the treatment of breast cancer. One such area of research is the use of PARP inhibitors in the TNBC population. Both PARP inhibitors and BRCA are both responsible for DNA damage repair. PARPs are responsible for single-stranded DNA repair, and BRCA is responsible for double-stranded DNA repair. In BRCA mutation carriers, when there is DNA damage to the tumor cells that cannot be repaired by BRCA because of a mutation, PARP repairs the DNA damage, thus allowing those tumor cells to grow and thrive. PARP inhibitors prevent DNA repair in tumor cells, leaving tumor cells without any mechanism for repair. This causes tumor cells to enter an apoptotic pathway leading to their demise. The use of PARP inhibitors BSI-021 and olaparib were the first 2 agents to be investigated and reported. A study of 74 patients treated with BSI-021 at 5.6 mg/kg combined with carboplatin and gemcitabine versus the same chemotherapeutic agents alone showed an increased objective response rate (48% versus 15%), increased PFS (3.3 to 6.9 months), increased clinical benefit (62% to 21%), and increased OS (5.7 to 9.2 months).[59] Similarly, in a phase II trial, the PARP inhibitor olaparib has been shown at a dose of 400 mg twice daily to improve PFS to 5.7 months with an overall response rate of 41%.[60,61] Currently, there are a number of ongoing clinical trials for various PARP inhibitors for BRCA mutation carriers in the neoadjuvant setting that hold exciting promise for this population with respect to local surgical treatment and OS.

### 3.11.2 *Vascular Endothelial Growth Factor (VEGF) Inhibitors*

Another area of ongoing research is the category of VEGF inhibitors. In the neoadjuvant setting, there are a number of trials open to patients with TNBC. Isakoff *et al.* used bevicizumab and cisplatin in the neoadjuvant setting in a triple-negative population and achieved a 16% pCR rate.[62] The Cancer and Leukemia Group B currently has an open trial, and the University of Tennessee Cancer Institute has a planned trial to examine the use of paclitaxil $\pm$ carboplatinum followed by AC $\pm$ bevicizumab in some combination for TNBC patients in the neoadjuvant setting. These trials should shed light on the question of whether a VEGF inhibitor improves pCR, and more importantly, whether a VEGF inhibitor improves DFS and OS.

While there are no trials currently open in the neoadjuvant setting examining a VEGF inhibitor for HER2-positive breast cancer, the BETH study (treatment of HER2-positive breast cancer with chemotherapy plus trastuzumab versus chemotherapy plus trastuzumab plus bevacizumab) will evaluate the efficacy of a VEGF inhibitor in the adjuvant setting. This trial is sponsored by the NSABP; if results are positive, this could lead to a neoadjuvant trial in the future.

In another area of research, there are alternative methods being evaluated using various predictive markers of pCR and survival. One such trial, the I-SPY, is open to HER2 positive and TNBC patients. In this trial, core biopsy specimens are obtained prior to chemotherapy, and various chemotherapeutic agents will be combined with novel therapies to assess tumor response. Similarly, a study sponsored by the United States Department of Defense is using core biopsy samples prior to NCT and subjecting them to chemo assays to obtain potential therapeutic response. This concept of personalizing breast cancer care based on tumor genomics prior to initiation of treatment will certainly play a large role in the way breast cancer is managed in the future. If more tumors can be obliterated with chemotherapy prior to surgery, more patients will be eligible for breast conservation and the OS of our patients may be greatly impacted.

## 3.12 Conclusion

The ultimate goal of NCT is to induce a complete pathologic response in the primary breast cancer and any involved lymph nodes. Not only does this render a patient eligible for BCS, but it also portents the best overall outcome for the breast cancer patient. Currently, to achieve this, one must consider the biological profile of the tumor and adjust chemotherapy regimens accordingly. In the future, however, there may be novel techniques which take into account the genomics of individual tumors, allowing a more personalized approach to treatment.

### 3.12.1 *Patient Vignettes*

#### 3.12.1.1 *Patient 1*

A 36-year-old woman presented with a palpable mass in her lateral right breast, which she detected on self-breast exam. The mammogram was negative for findings. A targeted ultrasound revealed a 3-cm solid mass in a B cup breast [Figure 3.1(a)]. Core needle biopsy revealed a triple-negative invasive ductal carcinoma. A clip was placed in the center of the mass at the time of core needle biopsy. A bilateral breast MRI revealed no other suspicious lesion in either breast [Figure 3.2(a)].

The patient desired breast conservation. Because she was going to receive adjuvant chemotherapy, she elected to have her chemotherapy in a neoadjuvant setting. This not only improved the likelihood of breast conservation but also improved her cosmetic outcome.

She underwent a sentinel node biopsy prior to start of chemotherapy, which was negative for metastatic disease, and was then given docetaxel, doxorubicin, and cyclophosphamide (TAC) 3-weekly for 6 cycles. She had a cCR to treatment. After repeating her ultrasound and MRI to evaluate response [Figures 3.1(b) and 3.2(b)], she underwent needle localized lumpectomy followed by whole breast radiation. Figure 3.3 shows the patient 6 months after completion of radiation treatment. Her pathology revealed no further invasive carcinoma, but residual atypical ductal

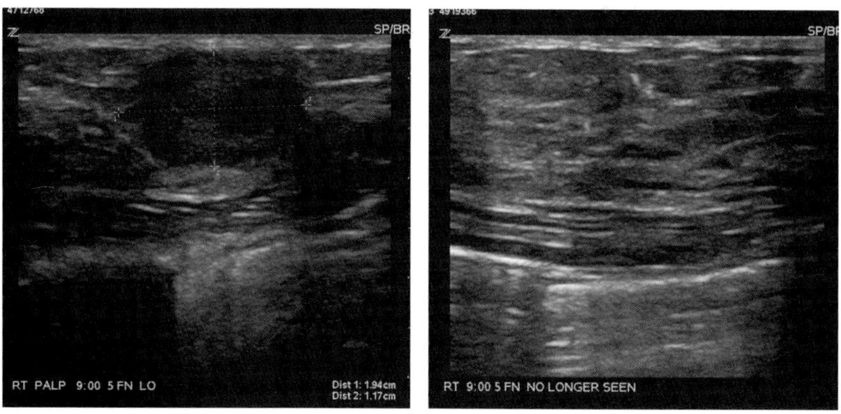


(a) (b)

Figure 3.1. (a) A 3-cm solid mass in a B-cup breast revealed by targeted ultrasound. (b) Repeated ultrasound to evaluate response.

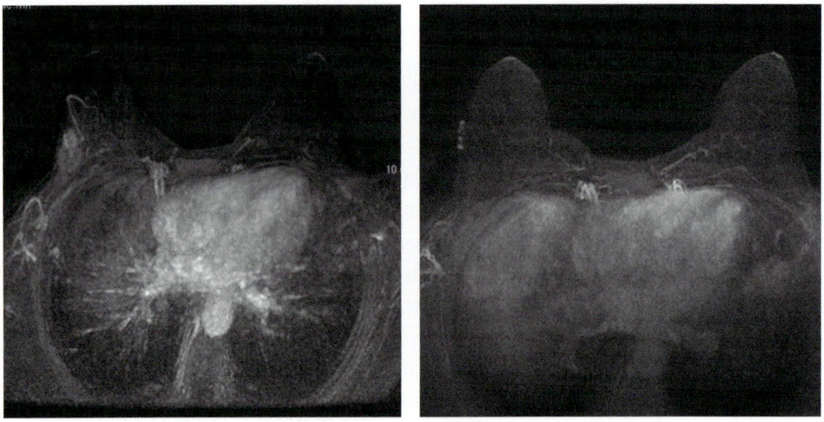

(a) (b)

Figure 3.2. (a) No other suspicious lesion in either breast revealed by bilateral breast MRI. (b) Repeated MRI to evaluate response.

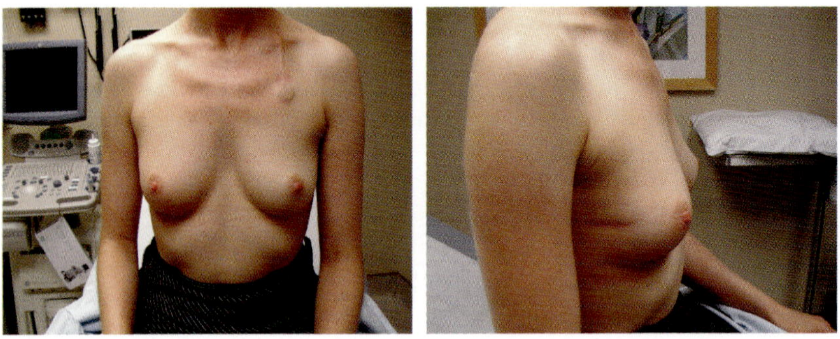

(a) (b)

Figure 3.3. Six months after completion of radiation treatment.

hyperplasia. The size of her surgical specimen was 4.5 cm × 3.5 cm × 1 cm. She remains disease free at 2 years.

#### 3.12.1.2 *Patient 2*

The patient, 50 years old, presented with a 5-cm mass in the UOQ of the right breast with N2 disease. Core needle biopsy confirmed the diagnosis of a triple-negative invasive ductal carcinoma, poorly differentiated with nodal metastasis. She was interested in breast preservation. Breast cup size: large B/small C.

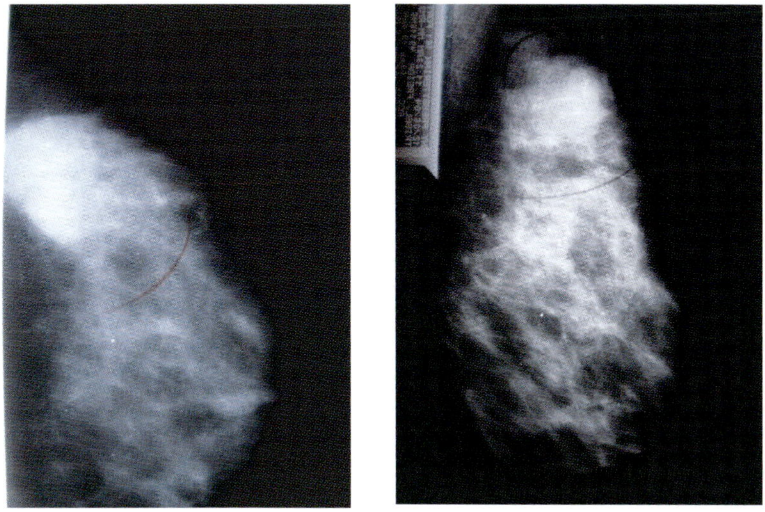

(a) (b)

Figure 3.4. Mammogram (a) pre-NCT and (b) post-NCT.

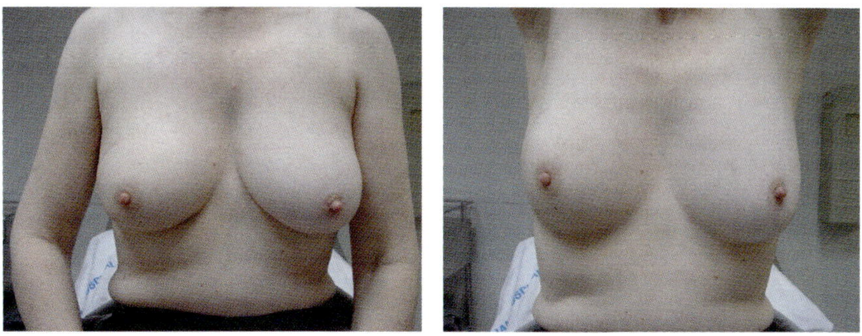

(a) (b)

Figure 3.5. Four years after completion of radiation therapy.

The patient received NCT (AC-T) with excellent clinical response. The first images show the mammogram pre- and post-NCT (Figure 3.4).

The patient underwent a lumpectomy and axillary node dissection with 2.5-cm residual disease in the breast. Figure 3.5 shows the patient 4 years after completion of radiation therapy.

## References


1. Fisher B, Anderson S, Bryant J, *et al.* (2002) Twenty-year follow-up of a randomized trial comparing total mastectomy, lumpectomy, and lumpectomy plus irradiation for the treatment of invasive breast cancer. *N Engl J Med* 347(16):1233–1241.
2. Perloff M, Lesnick GJ. (1982) Chemotherapy before and after mastectomy in stage III breast cancer. *Arch Surg* 117(7):879–881.
3. De Lena M, Zucali R, Viganotti G, *et al.* (1978) Combined chemotherapy-radiotherapy approach in locally advanced (T3b-T4) breast cancer. *Cancer Chemother Pharmacol* 1(1):53–59.
4. Rastogi P, Anderson SJ, Bear HD, *et al.* (2008) Preoperative chemotherapy: Updates of National Surgical Adjuvant Breast and Bowel Project Protocols B-18 and B-27. *J Clin Oncol* 26(5):778–785.
5. Sachelarie I, Grossbard ML, Chadha M, *et al.* (2006) Primary systemic therapy of breast cancer. *Oncologist* 11(6):574–589.
6. Mieog JS, van der Hage JA, van de Velde CJ. (2007) Neoadjuvant chemotherapy for operable breast cancer. *Br J Surg* 94(10):1189–1200.
7. Scholl SM, Fourquet A, Asselain B, *et al.* (1994) Neoadjuvant versus adjuvant chemotherapy in premenopausal patients with tumours considered too large for breast conserving surgery: Preliminary results of a randomised trial: S6. *Eur J Cancer* 30A(5):645–652.
8. Rouzier R, Mathieu MC, Sideris L, *et al.* (2004) Breast-conserving surgery after neoadjuvant anthracycline-based chemotherapy for large breast tumors. *Cancer* 101(5):918–925.
9. National Comprehensive Cancer Network Clinical Practice Guidelines: Breast Cancer. (2011) Version 2.2011.
10. Oh JL, Nguyen G, Whitman GJ, *et al.* (2007) Placement of radiopaque clips for tumor localization in patients undergoing neoadjuvant chemotherapy and breast conservation therapy. *Cancer* 110(11):2420–2427.
11. Whitman GJ, Strom EA. (2009) Workup and staging of locally advanced breast cancer. *Semin Radiat Oncol* 19(4):211–221.
12. Berg WA, Gilbreath PL. (2000) Multicentric and multifocal cancer: Whole-breast US in preoperative evaluation. *Radiology* 214(1):59–66.
13. Moon WK, Noh DY, Im JG. (2002) Multifocal, multicentric, and contralateral breast cancers: Bilateral whole-breast US in the preoperative evaluation of patients. *Radiology* 224(2):569–576.
14. Krishnamurthy S, Sneige N, Bedi DG, *et al.* (2002) Role of ultrasound-guided fine-needle aspiration of indeterminate and suspicious axillary lymph nodes in the initial staging of breast carcinoma. *Cancer* 95(5):982–988.
15. Shanta V, Swaminathan R, Rama R, Radhika R. (2008) Retrospective analysis of locally advanced noninflammatory breast cancer from Chennai, South India, 1990–1999. *Int J Radiat Oncol Biol Phys* 70(1):51–58.
16. Londero V, Bazzocchi M, Del Frate C, *et al.* (2004) Locally advanced breast cancer: Comparison of mammography, sonography and MR imaging in evaluation of residual disease in women receiving neoadjuvant chemotherapy. *Eur Radiol* 14(8):1371–1379.

17. Hylton N. (2006) MR imaging for assessment of breast cancer response to neoadjuvant chemotherapy. *Magn Reson Imaging Clin N Am* 14(3): 383–389, vii.
18. Le-Petross HC, Hylton N. (2010) Role of breast MR imaging in neoadjuvant chemotherapy. *Magn Reson Imaging Clin N Am* 18(2):249–258, viii–ix.
19. Loo CE, Teertstra HJ, Rodenhuis S, *et al.* (2008) Dynamic contrast-enhanced MRI for prediction of breast cancer response to neoadjuvant chemotherapy: Initial results. *AJR Am J Roentgenol* 191(5):1331–1338.
20. Zakhireh J, Gomez R, Esserman L. (2008) Converting evidence to practice: A guide for the clinical application of MRI for the screening and management of breast cancer. *Eur J Cancer* 44(18):2742–2752.
21. Houssami N, Hayes DF. (2009) Review of preoperative magnetic resonance imaging (MRI) in breast cancer: Should MRI be performed on all women with newly diagnosed, early stage breast cancer? *CA Cancer J Clin* 59(5):290–302.
22. Liedtke C, Mazouni C, Hess KR, *et al.* (2008) Response to neoadjuvant therapy and long-term survival in patients with triple-negative breast cancer. *J Clin Oncol* 26(8):1275–1281.
23. Carey LA, Dees EC, Sawyer L, *et al.* (2007) The triple negative paradox: Primary tumor chemosensitivity of breast cancer subtypes. *Clin Cancer Res* 13(8):2329–2334.
24. Wang S, Yang H, Tong F, *et al.* (2009) Response to neoadjuvant therapy and disease free survival in patients with triple-negative breast cancer. *Gan To Kagaku Ryoho* 36(2):255–258.
25. Garber JE, Richardson A, Harris LN, *et al.* (2006) Neoadjuvant cisplatin in "triple negative" breast cancer. *Breast Cancer Res Treat* 100:S149 (Abstract 3074).
26. Gronwald J, Byrski T, Huzarski T, *et al.* (2009) Neoadjuvant therapy with cisplatin in BRCA1-positive breast cancer patients. *J Clin Oncol* 27:15s (Abstract 502).
27. Buzdar AU, Ibrahim NK, Francis D, *et al.* (2005) Significantly higher pathologic complete remission rate after neoadjuvant therapy with trastuzumab, paclitaxel, and epirubicin chemotherapy: Results of a randomized trial in human epidermal growth factor receptor 2-positive operable breast cancer. *J Clin Oncol* 23(16):3676–3685.
28. Gianni L, Eiermann W, Semiglazov V, *et al.* (2010) Neoadjuvant chemotherapy with trastuzumab followed by adjuvant trastuzumab versus neoadjuvant chemotherapy alone, in patients with HER2-positive locally advanced breast cancer (the NOAH trial): A randomised controlled superiority trial with a parallel HER2-negative cohort. *Lancet* 375(9712):377–384.
29. Paluch-Shimon S, Wolf I, Goldberg H, *et al.* (2008) High efficacy of pre-operative trastuzumab combined with paclitaxel following doxorubicin & cyclophosphamide in operable breast cancer. *Acta Oncol* 47(8): 1564–1569.
30. Peintinger F, Buzdar AU, Kuerer HM, *et al.* (2008) Hormone receptor status and pathologic response of HER2-positive breast cancer treated with neoadjuvant chemotherapy and trastuzumab. *Ann Oncol* 19(12):2020–2025.

31. Straver ME, Rutgers EJ, Russell NS, *et al.* (2009) Towards rational axillary treatment in relation to neoadjuvant therapy in breast cancer. *Eur J Cancer* 45(13):2284–2292.
32. Mamounas EP. (2008) Facilitating breast-conserving surgery and preventing recurrence: Aromatase inhibitors in the neoadjuvant and adjuvant settings. *Ann Surg Oncol* 15(3):691–703.
33. Buzdar AU, Valero V, Theriault R, *et al.* (2003) Pathological complete response (pCR) to chemotherapy is related to hormone receptor status. *26th San Antonio Breast Cancer Symposium* (Abstract 302).
34. Tan MC, Al Mushawah F, Gao F, *et al.* (2009) Predictors of complete pathological response after neoadjuvant systemic therapy for breast cancer. *Am J Surg* 198(4):520–525.
35. Ellis MJ, Ma C. (2007) Letrozole in the neoadjuvant setting: The P024 trial. *Breast Cancer Res Treat* 105 (Suppl 1) 33–43.
36. Smith IE, Dowsett M, Ebbs SR, *et al.* (2005) Neoadjuvant treatment of postmenopausal breast cancer with anastrozole, tamoxifen, or both in combination: The Immediate Preoperative Anastrozole, Tamoxifen, or Combined with Tamoxifen (IMPACT) multicenter double-blind randomized trial. *J Clin Oncol* 23(22):5108–5116.
37. Howell A, Cuzick J, Baum M, *et al.* (2005) Results of the ATAC (Arimidex, Tamoxifen, Alone or in Combination) trial after completion of 5 years' adjuvant treatment for breast cancer. *Lancet* 365(9453):60–62.
38. Kurosumi M, Takatsuka Y, Watanabe T, *et al.* (2008) Histopathological assessment of anastrozole and tamoxifen as preoperative (neoadjuvant) treatment in postmenopausal Japanese women with hormone receptor-positive breast cancer in the PROACT trial. *J Cancer Res Clin Oncol* 134(6):715–722.
39. Barnadas A, Gil M, Gonzalez S, *et al.* (2009) Exemestane as primary treatment of oestrogen receptor-positive breast cancer in postmenopausal women: A phase II trial. *Br J Cancer* 100(3):442–449.
40. Mlineritsch B, Tausch C, Singer C, *et al.* (2008) Exemestane as primary systemic treatment for hormone receptor positive post-menopausal breast cancer patients: A phase II trial of the Austrian Breast and Colorectal Cancer Study Group (ABCSG-17). *Breast Cancer Res Treat* 112(1):203–213.
41. Takei H, Suemasu K, Inoue K, *et al.* (2008) Multicenter phase II trial of neoadjuvant exemestane for postmenopausal patients with hormone receptor-positive, operable breast cancer: Saitama Breast Cancer Clinical Study Group (SBCCSG-03). *Breast Cancer Res Treat* 107(1):87–94.
42. Tubiana-Hulin M, Becette V, Bieche I, *et al.* (2007) Exemestane as neoadjuvant hormonotherapy for locally advanced breast cancer: Results of a phase II trial. *Anticancer Res* 27(4C):2689–2696.
43. Akashi-Tanaka S, Shimizu C, Ando M, *et al.* (2009) 21-Gene expression profile assay on core needle biopsies predicts responses to neoadjuvant endocrine therapy in breast cancer patients. *Breast* 18(3):171–174.

44. Boughey JC, Wagner J, Garrett BJ, *et al.* (2009) Neoadjuvant chemotherapy in invasive lobular carcinoma may not improve rates of breast conservation. *Ann Surg Oncol* 16(6):1606–1611.
45. Bollet MA, Savignoni A, Pierga JY, *et al.* (2008) High rates of breast conservation for large ductal and lobular invasive carcinomas combining multimodality strategies. *Br J Cancer* 98(4):734–741.
46. Loibl S, von Minckwitz G, Raab G, *et al.* (2006) Surgical procedures after neoadjuvant chemotherapy in operable breast cancer: Results of the GEPARDUO trial. *Ann Surg Oncol* 13(11):1434–1442.
47. Regano S, Hernanz F, Ortega E, *et al.* (2009) Oncoplastic techniques extend breast-conserving surgery to patients with neoadjuvant chemotherapy response unfit for conventional techniques. *World J Surg* 33(10): 2082–2086.
48. Kirstein LJ, Rafferty E, Specht MC, *et al.* (2008) Outcomes of multiple wire localization for larger breast cancers: When can mastectomy be avoided? *J Am Coll Surg* 207(3):342–346.
49. Mamounas EP, Brown A, Anderson S, *et al.* (2005) Sentinel node biopsy after neoadjuvant chemotherapy in breast cancer: Results from National Surgical Adjuvant Breast and Bowel Project Protocol B-27. *J Clin Oncol* 23(12):2694–2702.
50. Kilbride KE, Lee MC, Nees AV, *et al.* (2008) Axillary staging prior to neoadjuvant chemotherapy for breast cancer: Predictors of recurrence. *Ann Surg Oncol* 15(11):3252–3258.
51. Krag DN, Anderson SJ, Julian TB, *et al.* (2007) Technical outcomes of sentinel-lymph-node resection and conventional axillary-lymph-node dissection in patients with clinically node-negative breast cancer: Results from the NSABP B-32 randomised phase III trial. *Lancet Oncol* 8(10):881–888.
52. Xing Y, Foy M, Cox DD, *et al.* (2006) Meta-analysis of sentinel lymph node biopsy after preoperative chemotherapy in patients with breast cancer. *Br J Surg* 93(5):539–546.
53. Sakakibara M, Nagashima T, Kadowaki M, *et al.* (2009) Clinical significance of axillary microresiduals after neoadjuvant chemotherapy in breast cancer patients with cytologically proven metastases. *Ann Surg Oncol* 16(9): 2470–2478.
54. Hunt KK, Yi M, Mittendorf EA, *et al.* (2009) Sentinel lymph node surgery after neoadjuvant chemotherapy is accurate and reduces the need for axillary dissection in breast cancer patients. *Ann Surg.*
55. Chen AM, Meric-Bernstam F, Hunt KK, *et al.* (2005) Breast conservation after neoadjuvant chemotherapy. *Cancer* 103(4):689–695.
56. Akay C, Meric-Bernstam F, Grubbs LG, *et al.* (2011) Validation of prognostic index score for local-regional recurrence after mastectomy or breast conservationtherapy in patients treated with NCT. *64th Annual Cancer Symposium*, Society Of Surgical Oncology, San Antonio TX (March 2011) (Abstract 34).

57. Fisher B, Bryant J, Wolmark N, *et al.* (1998) Effect of preoperative chemotherapy on the outcome of women with operable breast cancer. *J Clin Oncol* 16(8):2672–2685.
58. Kuerer HM, Newman LA, Smith TL, *et al.* (1999) Clinical course of breast cancer patients with complete pathologic primary tumor and axillary lymph node response to doxorubicin-based neoadjuvant chemotherapy. *J Clin Oncol* 17(2):460–469.
59. O'Shaughnessy JA, Osborne CK, Pippen JE, Jr., *et al.* (2009) Efficacy of BSI-201, a poly (ADP-ribose) polymerase-1 (PARP1) inhibitor, in combination with gemcitabine/carboplatin (G/C) in patients with metastatic triple-negative breast cancer (TNBC): Results of a randomized phase II trial. *J Clin Oncol* 27:18s (Abstract 3).
60. Fong PC, Boss DS, Carden CP, *et al.* (2008) AZD2281 (KU-0059436), a PARP (poly ADP-ribose polymerase) inhibitor with single agent anti-cancer activity in patients with BRCA deficient ovarian cancer: Results from a phase I study. *J Clin Oncol* 26 (Abstract 5510).
61. Yap TA, Boss DS, Fong PC, *et al.* (2007) First in human phase I pharmacokinetic (PK) and pharmacodynamic (PD) study of KU-0059436 (Ku), a small molecule inhibitor of poly ADP-ribose polymerase (PARP) in cancer patients (p), including BRCA1/2 mutation carriers. *J Clin Oncol* 25(18S): 3529.
62. Isakoff SJ. (2010) Triple-negative breast cancer: Role of specific chemotherapy agents. *Cancer J* 16(1):53–61.
63. Mauriac L, MacGrogan G, Avril A, *et al.* (1999) Neoadjuvant chemotherapy for operable breast carcinoma larger than 3 cm: A unicentre randomized trial with a 124-month median follow-up. Institut Bergonie Bordeaux Groupe Sein (IBBGS). *Ann Oncol* 10(1):47–52.
64. Rouzier R, Extra JM, Carton M, *et al.* (2001) Primary chemotherapy for operable breast cancer: Incidence and prognostic significance of ipsilateral breast tumor recurrence after breast-conserving surgery. *J Clin Oncol* 19(18):3828–3835.
65. Bonadonna G, Valagussa P, Brambilla C, *et al.* (1998) Primary chemotherapy in operable breast cancer: Eight-year experience at the Milan Cancer Institute. *J Clin Oncol* 16(1):93–100.
66. Chen AM, Meric-Bernstam F, Hunt KK, *et al.* (2004) Breast conservation after neoadjuvant chemotherapy: The MD Anderson Cancer Center. *J Clin Oncol* 22(12):2303–2312.
67. Cance WG, Carey LA, Calvo BF, *et al.* (2002) Long-term outcome of neoadjuvant therapy for locally advanced breast carcinoma: Effective clinical downstaging allows breast preservation and predicts outstanding local control and survival. *Ann Surg* 236(3):295–302 (Discussion 3).
68. Beriwal S, Schwartz GF, Komarnicky L, Garcia-Young JA. (2006) Breast-conserving therapy after neoadjuvant chemotherapy: Long-term results. *Breast J* 12(2):159–164.

# Chapter 4

# SKIN INCISIONS

Mahmoud El-Tamer

*Breast Service, Department of Surgery,
Memorial Sloan-Kettering Cancer Center,
New York, NY 10065, USA*

As of today, surgical resection remains the mainstay of breast cancer management. Multiple percutaneous and transcutaneous therapeutic modalities are currently being explored, but all remain experimental at this time. In order to achieve a surgical resection of a breast tumor, skin incisions remain mandatory. The long-term appearance of such incisions is crucial to the final cosmetic result. When planning an incision, the surgeon must keep multiple considerations in mind:

(1) Convenience for appropriate tumor removal
(2) Access to repair the defect
(3) Good cosmetic placement
(4) Allowance of further surgery (mastectomy without major inconvenience)

In the upper quadrants, we use curvilinear skin incisions most frequently. Curvilinear incisions placed in the lines of Kraissl[1] result in optimal healing and minimal scar separation. Furthermore, curvilinear incisions in the upper quadrant are optimal when resection of the tumor necessitates the removal of the overlying skin. After repair of an elliptical incision in the upper quadrant, the nipple areola is lifted, thereby enhancing the cosmetic result in a ptotic breast. Every effort should be made while designing the elliptical skin incision to avoid any displacement of the nipple, either laterally or medially. Misplacing the nipple areola complex may be more common in lesions that are on either side of the 12 o′clock axis.

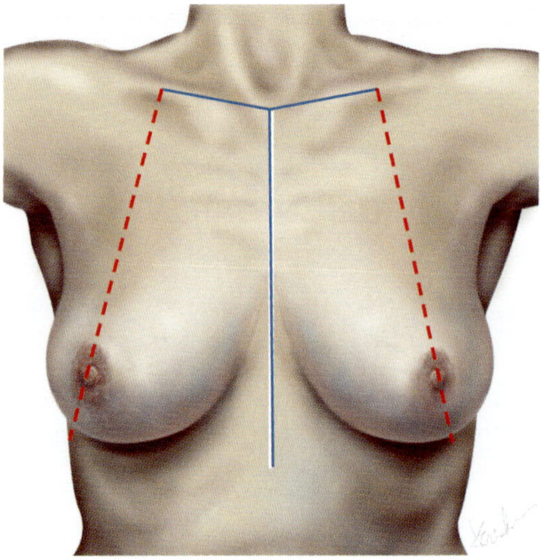

Figure 4.1. Guidance for appropriate nipple position.

We recommend that surgeons review the nipple meridian (Chapter 2) for guidance regarding the appropriate position of the nipple (Figure 4.1).

Excessive skin resection in the upper quadrant may result in the upward displacement of the nipple areola. We also try to avoid extending upper quadrant curvilinear incisions beyond the 3 o'clock and 9 o'clock axes. Such extensions may result in a suboptimal cosmetic result as scars traversing the 3 o'clock or 9 o'clock axes may widen or retract the NAC medially or laterally.

Radial incisions in the upper outer quadrant that are at the 10 o'clock axis on the right and the 2 o'clock axis on the left allow large resections of skin and underlying breast tissue with excellent repair. Such radial incisions may extend from the areolar edge up to the axilla, facilitating the performance of a sentinel node biopsy or even a complete axillary node dissection. Closure of these incisions does not usually result in the lateral retraction of the nipple areola complex. We limit radial incision in the upper outer quadrant to tumors that would otherwise require a quadrantectomy (Figure 4.2).[2]

Radial incisions can be performed in the upper inner quadrants of the breast. We believe, however, that they result in unsightly scars that are difficult to hide with a brassiere. We avoid placing any radial incisions between the 11 o'clock and 3 o'clock axes on the right side, and the 10 o'clock and 1 o'clock axes on the left (Figure 4.3).

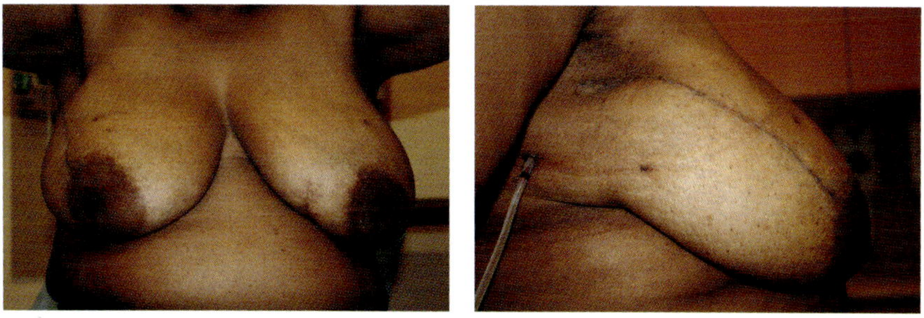

(a) (b)

Figure 4.2. Radial incision in the upper outer quadrant limited to tumors that would otherwise require a quadrantectomy.

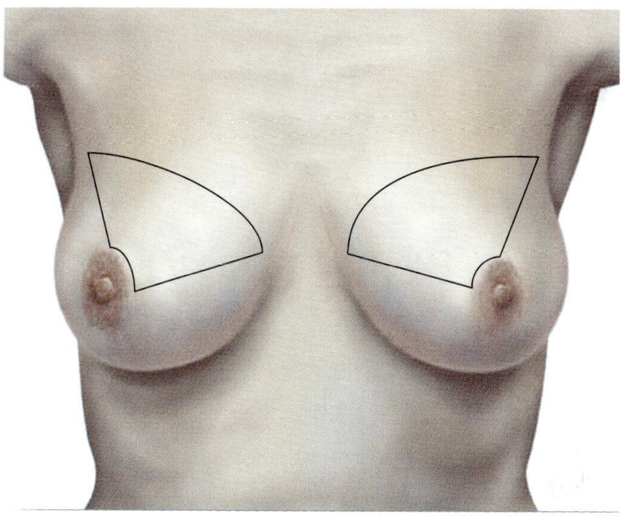

Figure 4.3. We avoid placing any radial incisions in the areas delineated in this drawing as they may result in unsightly scars.

In the lower quadrants, curvilinear incisions are applicable, particularly with small tumors. When the skin overlying a tumor is being excised as part of the resection, curvilinear incision should be avoided in the lower quadrants. Approximation of the skin after resection of a curvilinear elliptical skin incision in the lower quadrant will result in inferior displacement of the nipple areola and a corresponding unsatisfactory cosmetic appearance, better known as "Bird's Beak".[3] To avoid this type of cosmetic deformity, we use radial elliptical incision in the lower quadrants exclusively when

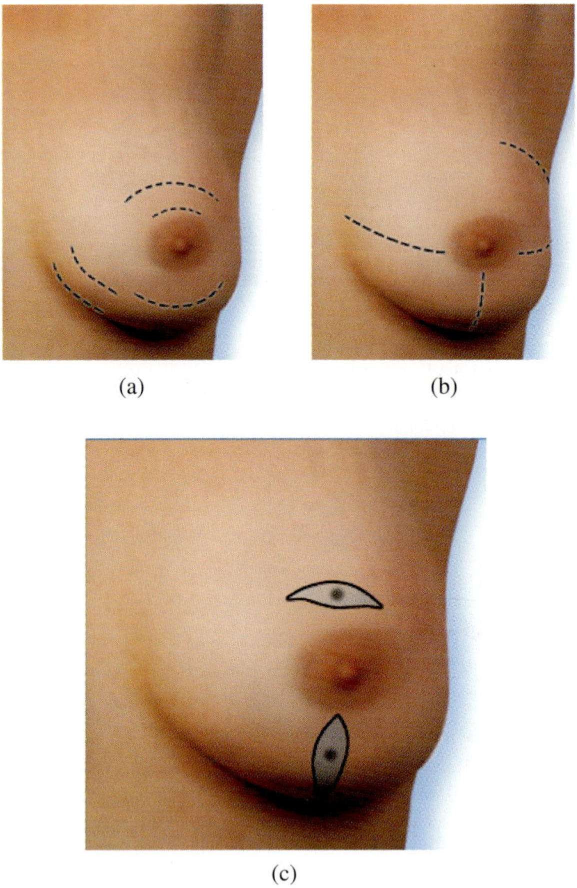


Figure 4.4. Radial incisions. (a) Curvilinear incision. (b) Radial incision. (c) Incision with skin excision.

planning skin resection. We also prefer radial incisions when faced with large-volume resection in the lower quadrants, as they facilitate repair of the defect in a mastopexy fashion, enhancing the final cosmetic outcome (Figure 4.4).

## 4.1 Periareolar Incision

In our experience, skin incisions performed around the areola provide the best cosmetic results. These wounds heal with minimal scarring, and due to

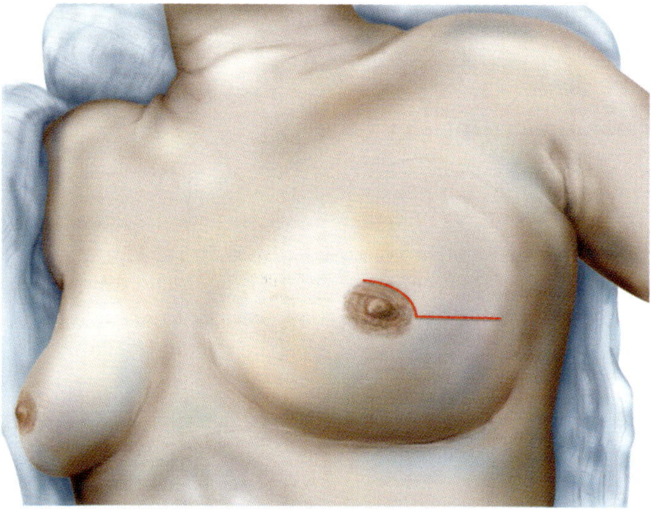

Figure 4.5. Periareolar incision.

their location, fade well, particularly when placed exactly at the edge of the areola. We recommend drawing the incision prior to prepping the patient because the edge of the areola may become blurry following painting with antiseptic solutions. This is particularly the case when using iodine-based solutions and in patients with fair skin tone coloring.

Areola size must be taken into consideration when planning periareolar incisions (Figure 4.5). Access to resection and repair may be limited in patients with areolar diameters of 2 cm or less. In this particular group, we recommend extending the incision laterally, medially, or both, at the 3 o′clock or 9 o′clock axes. Such extensions enhance access to and allow appropriate repair of the defect.

Maintaining the blood supply of the nipple areola complex during surgical intervention is crucial. We have rarely had any significant tissue loss with periareolar skin incisions, irrespective of the location of the incision, provided we have limited the skin incision to less than 50% of the circumference of the areola. During the surgical procedure, aggressive and prolonged retraction of the areola may result in significant damage to the blood supply, particularly in heavy smokers. We frequently release the traction on the areola to allow the flow of blood through the nipple areola complex. We also recommend judicious use of the electrocautery to the base of the nipple areola, particularly when the nipple areola complex is raised as a dermal flap. Patients frequently complain of loss of some of sensation with circumareolar incisions in the immediate perioperative period; however, the vast majority of patients report normal sensations 3 to 6 months after surgery.

## 4.2 Inframammary Incision

Incisions along the inframammary line have excellent cosmetic results, particularly in ptotic breasts. The scars are very well hidden, and patients frequently can only visualize the scars in a mirror. The scars allow good access to the breast and the possibility of utilizing the subcutaneous tissue below the inframammary line for reconstruction. One of the major inconveniences that arise with such incisions is their relative inconvenience when planning a completion mastectomy.

## 4.3 Skin Closure

We have made it a routine to approximate the skin in 2 layers, using absorbable suture. The first layer of closure is performed by approximating the deep dermis with interrupted and inverted 4-0 filaments. The sutures are applied at 1 cm to 2 cm intervals. We approximate the skin with running subcuticular 4-0 monofilament absorbable sutures. Dressing is accomplished with steri-strips with an overlying transparent impermeable adhesive. We always buttonhole the impermeable dressing to allow extrusion of the nipple (Figure 4.6).

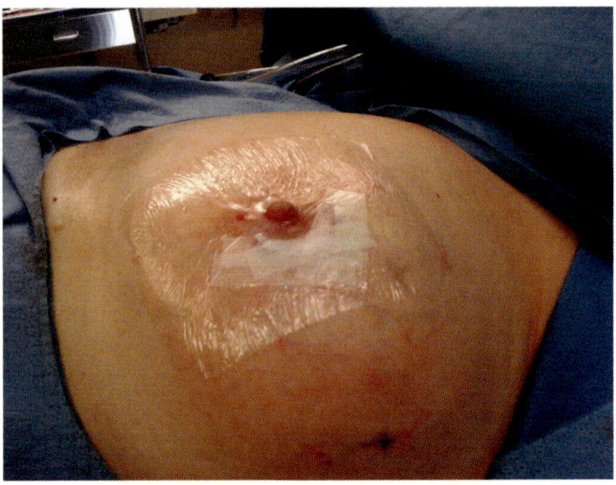

Figure 4.6. A buttonholed impermeable dressing allowing extrusion of the nipple.

## References

1. Kraissl CJ. (1951) The selection of appropriate lines for elective surgical incisions. *Plast Reconstr Surg (1946)* 8(1):1–28.
2. Veronesi U, Zurrida S. (2000) Quadrantectomy for malignant disease. *Operat Tech Gen Surg* 2:132–136.
3. Clough KB, Kaufman GJ, Nos C, *et al.* (2010) Improving breast cancer surgery: A classification and quadrant per quadrant atlas for oncoplastic surgery. *Ann Surg Oncol* 17(5):1375–1391.

# Chapter 5

# MARGINS IN BREAST CANCER SURGERY

Adriana D. Corben* and Monica Morrow†

**Department of Pathology,*
*Memorial Sloan-Kettering Cancer Center,*
*New York, NY10065, USA*

*†Breast Service, Department of Surgery,*
*Memorial Sloan-Kettering Cancer Center,*
*New York, NY10065, USA*

Breast-conserving therapy (BCT), consisting of the removal of the primary tumor and whole breast irradiation, is a well-accepted method for breast cancer management. Six prospective randomized trials, some with follow-up of 20 years or more,[1,2] have established without a doubt that there is no survival advantage for mastectomy compared with the more limited surgery and radiation therapy (RT). Over time, the rates of local recurrence after BCT have declined steadily and are now considerably less than 10% at 10 years of follow-up.[3,4] However, the appropriate extent of surgical resection needed to maintain local control remains a matter of debate, and the lack of consensus regarding what constitutes an adequate negative margin results in multiple trips to the operating room for margin re-excision in a significant number of patients, and unnecessary mastectomies in others.[5] The perception that a more widely clear margin enhances local control has been a major factor in the development of oncoplastic surgery.

The demonstration in the Early Breast Cancer Trialists Collaborative Group (EBCTCG) overview that differences in local control between treatments of 10%–20% at 5 years are associated with significant differences in breast cancer-specific survival at 15 years[6] has focused new attention on the importance of local control. For many years, disease burden as defined by margin status was felt to be the primary determinant of local control. Over time, it has become increasingly clear that both the underlying genetics of the tumor and the availability of effective systemic therapy are also critical components of local control. In this chapter, we will discuss techniques of margin evaluation, review the available data on the relationship between margin status and local control for invasive and intraductal cancer, and discuss the impact of molecular subtype of breast cancer and targeted therapy on local control outcomes.

## 5.1 Methods of Margin Evaluation

The term "margin" is often used without specifying the pathologic method used to determine the margin status. Unfortunately, there is neither a standard method of margin evaluation nor a standard number of histologic sections that are examined from each margin surface. Margins can be evaluated using a radial method, shaved method, or by shaving the walls of the lumpectomy cavity. These techniques are described later. Variations in pathology protocols take on considerable potential significance when clinicians assert that differences of 1–2 mm separate an adequate from an inadequate resection. This variability in margin processing is documented in a study which examined 91 consecutive excisional breast biopsies submitted from 50 different hospitals to a single university pathology department over a 2-year period.[7] Only 18% of reports described the technique (shaved or radial) used to evaluate the margins. Only 30% of the specimens were submitted in total; an unknown amount of tissue was submitted in 1%, and representative sections averaging 13 blocks per specimen were submitted in 69%.

### 5.1.1 *Radial Margin Approach*

The most common method of margin assessment is the perpendicular (or radial) margin technique, which allows for precise measurement of the distance separating the tumor from the inked margin. With this method, the specimen is received with at least 2 of the margins marked with clips or sutures to allow specimen orientation. The 6 margins of the specimen are inked in 6 different colors by the prosector. The ink should be applied gently so that no artificial disruption occurs. Excess ink should be carefully removed by pressing with gauze to reduce the problem of "running" ink. A brief application of acetone on the inked surface helps stain enhancement and reduces the problem of running ink. The inked specimen is sequentially cut into 0.2–0.3 cm slices, perpendicular to its long axis, so that the

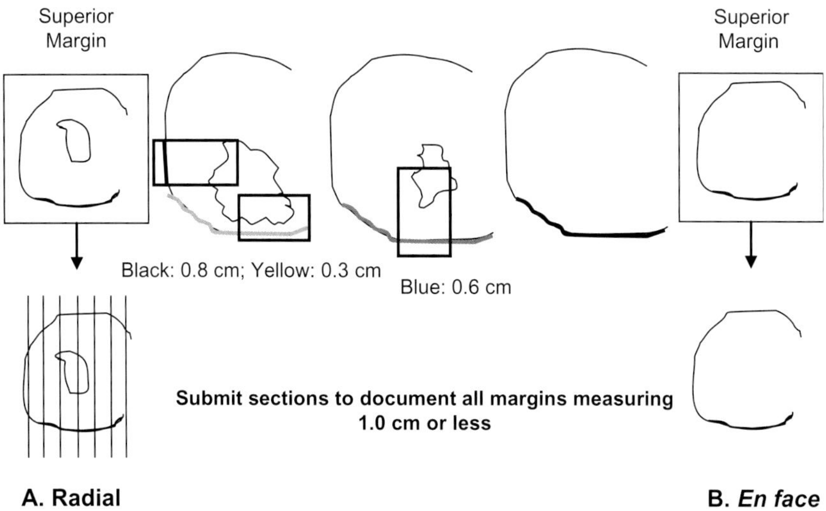


Figure 5.1. (a) Radial (perpendicular) margin evaluation. With the radial margin technique, each margin surface is inked a different color, and the distance from the tumor to the ink is reported for each margin. (b) Shaved (*en face*) margin evaluation. With the *en face* method, the entire surface is shaved and no inking is needed.

perimeter of each tissue slice contains a few (2 to 4) margins identified by the different ink colors. Margins within 0.5 cm from the index lesion are best evaluated in their entirety, and the more distant margins can be representatively sampled [Figure 5.1(a)]. With this method, the pathologist can report the exact microscopic distance from the tumor to each individual margin and distinguish between a truly positive margin (tumor at ink) and a close margin. The extent of tumor at the margin or in close proximity to it can also be assessed.

The disadvantages of this method include running ink, imprecise margin orientation, and surface complexity. Running of the ink from the irregular fatty specimen surface to the inside of the specimen [Figure 5.2(a)], and different color inks running into each other [Figure 5.2(b)], occur frequently, leading to possible overinterpretation and false-positive margins. In addition, the breast tissue is soft and may be artificially disrupted when the specimen is compressed to obtain a specimen radiograph or during gross examination. The flattening of the specimen in the gross room may distort the margin orientation. In one study, surgeons and pathologists disagreed on margin designation in 31% of cases when 2 marking sutures for orientation were placed in the operating room. The presence of skin or muscle on the specimen did not reduce the disorientation rate, but the specimen size was highly correlated with this problem. Specimens less than 20 cm in size

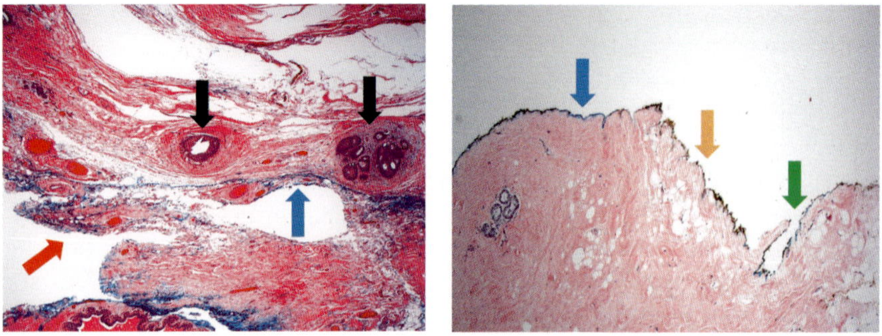

(a) (b)

Figure 5.2. Problems with radial margin assessment and inking. (a) "Running" of ink (blue arrow) inside a specimen challenges the interpretation of the distance of the ductal carcinoma *in situ* (black arrows) from the true inked resection margin (red arrow). (b) Different color inks (orange, blue and green arrows) running into each other create false interpretations of margin designation.

had a disorientation rate of 78% compared to only 20% for larger specimens ($p < 0.001$).[8] In addition, it has been estimated that the complete examination of a 2 cm spherical specimen would require in excess of 3,000 sections.[9] Taking into account that the surfaces of breast excisions are highly complex and irregular, and that the surface area of some specimens is quite large, margin assessment, using the inked radial margin method, is highly subject to sampling error.

### 5.1.2 *Shaved Margin Approach*

The use of shaved (*en face*) margins allows the oriented specimen to be inked entirely in one color as long as the prosector is able to maintain the proper orientation. This eliminates the problem of different colored inks running together. The margins are shaved off parallel to the outer surface of the specimen, similar to the process of peeling an orange, at a tissue depth of 0.2–0.3 cm [Figure 5.1(b)]. The shaved margins closest to the index lesion are submitted entirely. The sections are embedded *en face* with the inked surface facing downward so that the microscopic examination starts from the inner aspect of the tissue. With this method, a margin is reported as positive when the tumor is present anywhere in the section. This means that malignant cells may be present within a 0.2–0.3 cm radius from the surgical margin or at the margin itself, but that the exact distance of the tumor to margin cannot be assessed. If no tumor is identified, the margin is reported as negative. The advantages of this method include a straightforward microscopic examination, no occurrence of ink problems, and the examination of a large proportion of the specimen's surface with relatively few sections. Although advantageous to the pathologist, this technique is extremely problematic for surgeons because it substantially increases the number of margins which are called positive.

Guidi *et al.*[10] compared the shaved margin technique with the conventional radial margin method by evaluating 22 surgical specimens using both methods. The specimens were inked, and the margins were shaved and microscopically examined. The tissue was then extracted from the block, cut perpendicular to the inked surface, and re-embedded to assess the radial inked margin status. The study demonstrated that a negative shaved margin was highly predictive of a negative inked margin (98% concordance), but the positive predictive value was much lower, with only 61% of the positive shaved margins being called positive (tumor at ink) by the radial margin technique. In a study at Memorial Sloan-Kettering Cancer Center (MSKCC), Wright *et al.* reported that when the MSKCC Department of Pathology switched from radial margin assessment to the shaved method, the positive margin rate increased from 16% to 49% even though the surgical technique did not change.[11]

### 5.1.3 *Cavity Shave Approach*

The evaluation of separate cavity shaves, obtained by the surgeon, provides a solution to margin assessment which combines the advantages of both the radial and the shaved margins. With this approach (Figure 5.3), the surgeon resects the index lesion and then takes separate shaved margins from the surgical cavity. A separate anterior margin may or may not be submitted. The main specimen, containing the tumor, is received unoriented and does not necessarily need to be inked. The tumor is entirely sampled, including any prior biopsy site, and 1 or 2 representative sections of any grossly uninvolved breast tissue present are also submitted. Each shave specimen represents a margin (medial, lateral, inferior, superior, and posterior walls of the surgical cavity) and is received oriented with a suture or metal clip, designating the final margin surface. Sometimes, one specimen may consist of 2 adjacent margins. Each margin is inked on the side designated by the suture or clip, perpendicularly sectioned, and submitted either entirely or representatively in 10 blocks (Figure 5.3). In our institution, after an internal review, only 6 blocks are now submitted per shave specimen unless any epithelial atypia or carcinoma is microscopically identified; the remaining margin is then entirely submitted. This technique allows precise margin designation and accurate measurement of the margin width. These specimens

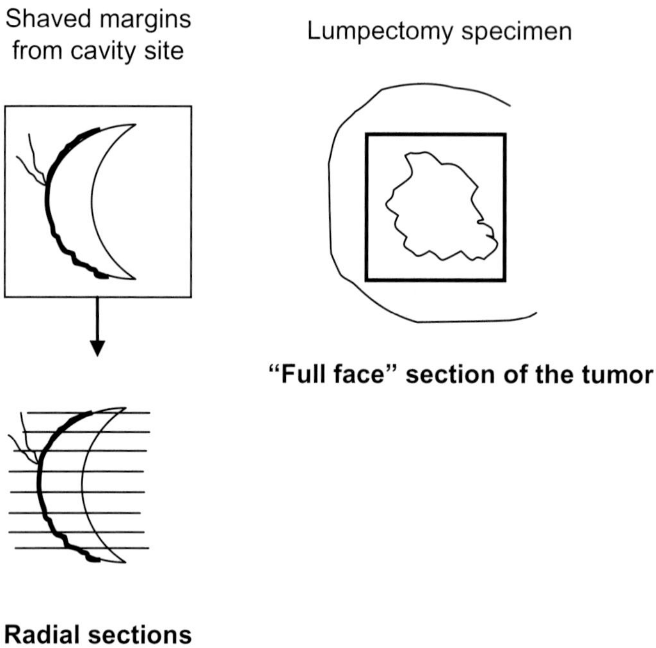


Figure 5.3. Cavity shaved margin evaluation (1 out of 5 shown). With the cavity margin evaluation method, the primary lumpectomy specimen is not inked. The outer surface of each of the individual margins is inked, and the distance to any tumor measured.

are more easily handled by the prosector with limited manipulation of the tissue, and the use of the same color ink contributes to a reduction of problematic artifacts of the prior described techniques. A significant increase in the number of blocks and slides is the main disadvantage of this method for most institutions. A number of investigators have reported that this method significantly reduces the rate of re-excision for close margins.[12–18] These results are summarized in Table 5.1. One issue with the routine use of cavity shave margins is the potential removal of larger amounts of breast tissue, resulting in a worsening of cosmetic outcome. Huston *et al.* compared the rates of margin positivity and volume of tissue, excised among patients undergoing lumpectomy, with shaving of all margins ($n = 45$), lumpectomy with selective shaving of margins thought by the surgeon to be suspicious ($n = 77$), and lumpectomy alone ($n = 49$). The routine resection of additional margins resulted in the lowest re-operation rate, 17.7%, compared to 32.5% and 38.7% for selective re-excision and lumpectomy, respectively. The mean total specimen volumes were 129 cm,$^3$ 46 cm,$^3$ and 37 cm$^3$ for the 3 groups.[12] In contrast,

Table 5.1. Impact of tumor cavity sampling on re-excision rates.

| Author | # Cases | % Positive margin: Cavity margins | % Positive margin: Routine | $P$-value |
|---|---|---|---|---|
| Huston TL[12] | 171 | 18 | 39 | |
| Jacobson AF[13] | 125 | 18 | 66 | |
| Tengher-Barna I[17] | 107 | 13 | 33 | |
| Marudanayagam R[15] | 786 | 5.6 | 12.5 | <0.01 |
| Rizzo M[16] | 320 | 15 | 43 | <0.05 |
| Kobberman A[14] | 138 | 22 | 42 | 0.01 |

Rizzo *et al.*[16] found no difference in the volume removed with or without additional shaved margins if negative margins were achieved with the initial excision. However, in patients requiring re-excision, a smaller total volume of breast tissue was removed if the cavity shave technique was used initially ($p < 0.005$).

### 5.1.4 *Other Issues Related to Margin Assessment*

In addition to the method of margin assessment, other factors related to specimen processing may influence the margin width or whether or not the tumor is identified at the margin. Graham *et al.* compared the measurement of the mean height of the lumpectomy specimen in the operating room by the surgeon to the measurement in the pathology lab in 100 consecutive specimens[19] and found a 46% decrease from a mean of 2.6 cm as measured by the surgeon to 1.4 cm as measured in pathology. This was independent of patient age, lesion type (mass versus calcifications) or breast density. When compression devices were used for specimen radiography, the decrease was 54% compared to 41% when these devices were not used ($p = 0.0003$). These findings indicate that measurements of anterior and posterior margin distances on the primary tumor specimen are subject to significant variation depending upon how the specimen is handled.

## 5.2 Margin Width and Local Recurrence: Invasive Cancer

Considering the lack of standardization in pathology methods, it is not surprising that there is little consensus regarding what constitutes an adequate negative margin. Azu *et al.*[20] surveyed a population-based sample of 318 surgeons identified from patients in the Surveillance, Epidemiology, and End Results (SEER) registry. Surgeons were asked "What negative margin width precludes the need for re-excision in a 60-year-old with a 0.8 cm invasive cancer which is estrogen receptor (ER), progesterone receptor (PR), and HER2 negative?" The following four options were offered: Tumor not touching ink; >1–2 mm; >5 mm; or >10 mm. No answer was endorsed by more than 50% of respondents. Only 11% selected the tumor not touching ink option, 42% selected >1–2 mm, and 19% selected >10 mm. Similar variation exists among radiation oncologists. In a survey of 1,133 North American and European radiation oncologists, 45% of those from North America endorsed a margin of tumor not touching ink, while those in Europe favored more widely clear margins, with greater than 5 mm being the most common answer, selected by 29%.[21] The lack of consensus on what constitutes an adequate negative margin results in the frequent performance of re-excision to obtain more widely clear margins. Morrow *et al.*,[5] reporting on a population-based sample from the SEER registry of 800 women attempting BCT, observed that although the procedure was successful in 88%, 22% underwent a re-excision. Other studies report a wide variation in re-excision rates ranging from 6%[15] to 49%,[22] with the majority noting re-excision in 15% to 30% of patients.[12,23,24]

The prospective randomized trials that established the safety and efficacy of BCT[1,2,25–28] do not provide much guidance on the margin question because only the National Surgical Adjuvant Breast and Bowel Project (NSABP) B06 trial used a microscopic definition of a negative margin, which was tumor not touching ink.[1] Although the other trials are often perceived as requiring more widely clear margins, they relied upon gross margin definitions, making the actual margin width impossible to assess. Similarly, although a trial by Veronesi *et al.*, which randomized patients to quadrantectomy or a more limited tumorectomy, demonstrated a lower rate of local recurrence in the quadrantectomy group (2.2% versus 7.0%), this study also relied on gross margin assessment. The tumorectomy was performed with a gross margin of 1 cm, but in a subset of patients who had microscopic margin evaluation, 16% of those in the tumorectomy group had positive margins.[29] The uncertainty over margin status in this trial makes it impossible to conclude that a larger quadrantectomy-type procedure is associated with a lower rate of local recurrence than a more limited resection with negative inked margins. The authors have been unable to identify any prospective randomized trials that directly compare outcomes between microscopically verified margins of differing widths.

Recently, Houssami *et al.* performed a methodologically rigorous meta-analysis of the relationship between local recurrence and margin distance.[30]

The analysis included 21 studies with 14,571 patients and 1,026 local recurrences. The relationship between margin status and local recurrences was verified, with an odds ratio (OR) for local recurrence of 2.42 for positive versus negative margins ($p < 0.001$). No relationship between margin width, defined as 1 mm versus 2 mm versus 5 mm, and local recurrence was identified. Although a trend for a benefit of more widely clear margins was seen in some models, this was not statistically significant after adjusting for other treatment factors, such as the use of a radiation boost or receipt of endocrine therapy. This meta-analysis, which included information on a large number of factors relevant to local recurrences, such as date of study enrollment, patient age, use of radiation including a boost, and pathologic tumor features such as lymphovascular invasion (LVI), extensive intraductal component (EIC), and tumor grade, provides the most convincing evidence to date that margins more widely clear than tumor not touching ink do not have a major impact upon local control in the era of modern multidisciplinary therapy.

Although this may seem counterintuitive, it becomes much more logical if one considers that even mastectomy does not eliminate the problem of local recurrence. In the initial randomized trials comparing BCT to mastectomy in which at least grossly negative margins were required, only the Milan study,[2] which included T1 cancers treated with radical mastectomy, showed a statistically significant reduction in local recurrence for mastectomy compared to BCT (Table 5.2).[1,25,26] This, coupled with the observation from the EBCTCG overview[6] that even with the addition of postmastectomy RT, the incidence of local recurrence is higher in node-positive women than it is in node-negative women, indicates that local recurrence may be due to either excessive tumor burden or aggressive biology. The failure to observe a decrease in local recurrence with surgical margins more widely clear than tumor on ink suggests that once the disease burden is reduced to this level (i.e., no clinically detectable cancer), tumor biology is the main determinant of local control.

Table 5.2. Local recurrence in randomized trials of mastectomy versus BCT.

| | | % Local recurrence | |
|---|---|---|---|
| Trial | Follow-up (yrs) | BCT | Mastectomy |
| Institute Gustave-Roussy[25] | 15 | 9 | 14 |
| Milan 1[2] | 20 | 9 | 2* |
| NSABP B06[1] | 20 | 14 | 10 |
| Danish[26] | 6 | 3 | 4 |

*$p < 0.0001$. BCT, breast-conserving therapy.

### 5.2.1 *The Influence of Histology on Margin Width*

Variations in the growth patterns of different histologic types of cancers raise the possibility that the same margin width may not be appropriate for all histologic tumor types. Infiltrating lobular cancers are frequently multifocal and grow as single cells in linear strands separated by normal stroma,[31] raising the possibility that margins negative only by "tumor not touching ink" might be associated with a significant residual tumor burden. However, clinical studies do not document a higher rate of local recurrence after BCT for lobular cancers compared to ductal cancers,[32–34] suggesting that if negative margins are obtained, the growth pattern is irrelevant. Galimberti *et al.*[35] analyzed 382 patients with pure infiltrating lobular carcinoma, treated with BCT, to determine if rates of local control differed among those with margins less than 1 cm compared to 1 cm or greater. The local failure rate was 4.6% for the less than 1 cm margin group compared to 3.7% in the 1 cm or greater group, leading the authors to conclude that more widely negative margins were not necessary for patients with infiltrating lobular carcinoma.

The other group of concern is patients with an EIC in association with their invasive cancer. Early studies, performed prior to the routine inking of margins, suggested that an EIC was associated with higher rate of local recurrence in patients undergoing BCT.[36] Holland *et al.* documented that approximately 30% of patients with EIC-positive cancers had prominent intraductal carcinoma more than 2 cm beyond the primary tumor, compared to only 2% of patients with EIC-negative tumors,[37] indicating that a substantial number of patients with an EIC, treated by excision to grossly negative margins, have a heavy residual tumor burden. When patients with an EIC are excised to negative-inked margins, the rates of local recurrence are not increased compared with patients without an EIC.[38,39] However, Faverly *et al.* have demonstrated that low- and intermediate-grade ductal carcinoma *in situ* (DCIS) often grows with gaps between the DCIS lesions, although these gaps are usually less than 5 mm in size,[40] suggesting that margins negative by only tumor not touching ink could be associated with a significant residual tumor burden. The issue of margins and DCIS is discussed in detail later in this chapter. The presence of an EIC in association with invasive cancer indicates it may be prudent to obtain a margin of at least 2 mm if large amounts of DCIS are in proximity to the margin. In the case of both infiltrating lobular carcinoma and an EIC, clinical judgment remains important. A single duct of DCIS or microscopic focus of lobular carcinoma in close proximity to the margin is unlikely to be associated with a heavy residual tumor burden, whereas a large area of tumor immediately adjacent to a margin is associated with a greater risk of residual disease[41] and should prompt re-excision.

### 5.2.2 *Other Factors Influencing Local Control in Invasive Cancer*

It is important to recognize that a "negative" margin does not indicate that there is no residual tumor in the breast. Holland *et al.*,[42] in a landmark study using serial subgross sectioning to evaluate the remaining breast tissue in 264 mastectomy specimens from patients with clinically unifocal cancers 4 cm or less in size, showed that only 39% of cases had no additional tumor beyond the index cancer. In 20% of cases the tumor foci were within 2 cm of the index tumor, and in 41% of cases the tumor foci were more than 2 cm from the primary tumor (Figure 5.4). From a practical point of view, a negative margin indicates that the residual tumor burden in the breast is low enough that it is likely to be controlled by RT. The role of RT in maintaining local control is well documented in the EBCTCG overview.[6] At 5 years, the absolute incidence of local recurrence in node-negative women receiving RT was 16% lower than in those not receiving RT, while a 30% reduction in isolated local recurrence was seen for node-positive women. These reductions in local recurrence at 5 years translate to 15-year survival gains of 5% and 7% in node-negative and node-positive women, respectively. Bartelink *et al.*, in a prospective randomized trial examining the benefits of boost dose of RT on local control, demonstrated statistically significant reductions in local recurrence with the addition of a boost in women of all ages.[43] While the role of RT in local control has long been recognized, the impact on local control of both improvements in systemic therapy and its widespread use are less well recognized.

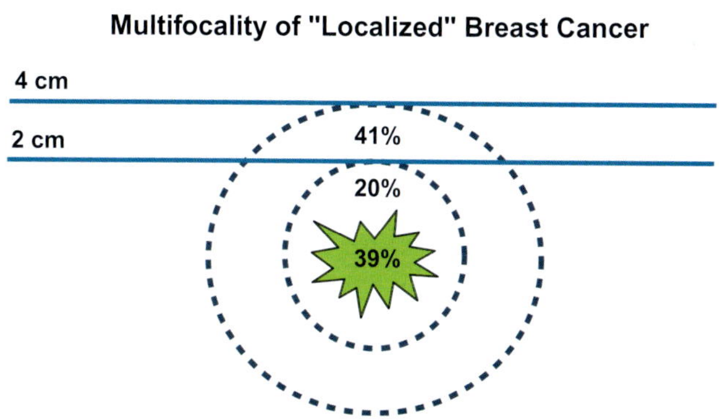


Figure 5.4. Distribution of cancer identified on serial subgross sectioning of 264 mastectomy specimens with clinically localized tumors less than 4 cm in size. Only 39% of clinically localized cancers had all malignant cells confined to the tumor mass. In 20% of the cases, the residual cancer was within 2 cm of the primary; in the remainder, it was within 4 cm. (Data from Holland R *et al.*[42])

The majority of women with invasive breast cancer now receive some form of adjuvant systemic therapy in addition to surgery and RT. Both endocrine therapy and chemotherapy significantly reduce the likelihood of local recurrence after BCT. In the NSABP B14 trial, in which node-negative, ER positive women were randomized to tamoxifen citrate or placebo, the 10-year rate of in-breast recurrence was reduced from 14.7% in the placebo group to 4.3% in the tamoxifen group.[44] In the NSABP B13 trial, node-negative ER negative women were randomized to chemotherapy or a no-treatment control group.[45] At 8 years, local recurrence was seen in only 2.6% of those receiving chemotherapy compared with 13.4% of controls. In a report of 3,799 node-negative women participating in 5 NSABP trials of adjuvant systemic therapy, the cumulative incidence of in-breast recurrence at 12 years for those receiving adjuvant therapies was only 6.6%.[3] Since the time that these trials were conducted, our ability to target therapy has improved, and this will undoubtedly result in a further decrease in local recurrence rates. For example, in the randomized trials that established the efficacy of adjuvant trastuzumab, the addition of trastuzumab to chemotherapy resulted in a 40% decrease in locoregional recurrence compared to treatment with chemotherapy alone.[46] Similar results have been reported in ER positive, node-negative patients when systemic treatment is selected on the basis of the Oncotype Dx™ score. Although this score was developed to predict the risk of systemic recurrence, Mamounas *et al.*[47] demonstrated that in the absence of systemic treatment, patients with high-risk Oncotype Dx™ scores had an 18.4% risk of locoregional recurrence (LRR) compared to those with low-risk scores who had a 10.8% risk. The addition of tamoxifen, appropriate treatment for those with low-risk scores, reduced the incidence of LRR by more than 50% to 4.3% in the low-risk group. In contrast, a much more modest reduction in LRR from 18.4% to 15.8% was seen in the high-risk group. However, when chemotherapy was added, the LRR rate in the high-risk group decreased to 7.8%.

The importance of biology and targeted therapy is further supported by the emerging literature on the impact of tumor subtype on local recurrence after BCT or mastectomy. Both Millar *et al.*[48] and Nguyen *et al.*[49] have demonstrated that the rate of local recurrence after BCT varies among the intrinsic subtypes of breast cancer as approximated by ER, PR, and HER2 status. In both studies, the lowest rates of local recurrence at 5 years were seen among the ER, PR positive, HER2-negative (Luminal A-like) group, and the highest rates among the triple negative (basal-like) and ER negative, HER2-positive patients in the absence of adjuvant trastuzumab. However, ER, PR, and HER2 status are not indicators of the need for more widely clear margins because the same pattern of an increased risk of chest wall recurrence among ER negative patients, regardless of HER2 status, was observed in a retrospective analysis of the Danish Breast Cancer Group randomized trials of mastectomy with or without RT.[50] As previously noted, the addition of trastuzumab to chemotherapy has been shown to reduce the risk of local recurrence in HER2-overexpressing patients,[46] indicating that targeted therapy is a major contributor to local control. In aggregate, this information indicates that factors other than disease burden are key determinants of local control.

### 5.2.3 *Margins After Neoadjuvant Chemotherapy*

Prospective randomized trials have demonstrated that the use of preoperative (neoadjuvant) chemotherapy allows BCT in patients who would have required a mastectomy if surgery was performed initially.[51,52] A meta-analysis of randomized trials of neoadjuvant versus adjuvant chemotherapy demonstrated no increase in the risk of LRR after neoadjuvant therapy as long as surgery was performed (hazard ratio, 1.12; 95% confidence interval (CI), 0.92–1.37; $p = 0.25$).[53] However, in the NSABP B18 trial, after 9 years of follow-up, the patients who required chemotherapy to downstage to lumpectomy ($n = 65$) had a 15.9% rate of in-breast recurrence compared to 9.9% for those who were lumpectomy candidates at presentation ($p = 0.04$).[54] This finding raises the possibility that margins need to be considered somewhat differently in the setting of neoadjuvant therapy.

The purpose of neoadjuvant therapy is to allow the removal of a smaller amount of breast tissue than would be necessary if initial surgery was performed. Breast cancer shrinkage in response to neoadjuvant therapy has been shown to occur in 2 different ways: concentrically, and in a honeycomb or buckshot pattern. MRI is the most reliable means of assessing both the amount of residual tumor and the pattern of shrinkage.[55] In patients with a pathologic complete response or concentric tumor shrinkage, the consideration of margin width does not differ from that in the primary surgical setting. In patients with the honeycomb pattern, the determination of the appropriate extent of resection is more problematic. Investigators from the University of Texas MD Anderson Cancer Center have shown that on multivariate analysis, a honeycomb pattern of response, residual disease >2 cm, and clinical N2 or N3 disease were statistically significant predictors of local recurrence after BCT.[56] However, whether the higher rate of local recurrence observed with the honeycomb pattern of shrinkage can be reduced with more widely clear margins is uncertain because this pattern of shrinkage may be a reflection of biologic properties of the tumor which influence local recurrence just as they do in the primary surgical setting. Evidence supporting this concept comes from a study of 149 patients examining the impact of ER, PR, and HER2 status on local recurrence after neoadjuvant therapy.[57] The highest rate of local recurrence was seen in the ER, PR, and HER2-negative group, just as was seen in studies examining the significance of these markers in the primary surgical setting.[48,49] In the absence of definitive information on the benefit of more widely clear margins after neoadjuvant therapy, it seems prudent to follow the current joint guideline of the American College of Surgeons, American College of Radiology, and College of American Pathologists which suggests that if viable resident tumor is present scattered throughout the lumpectomy specimen, even if it is not actually on the margin, re-excision should be considered.[58]

### 5.2.4 *Summary and Conclusions: Invasive Cancer*

The failure of mastectomy, the most widely clear margin which can be obtained in the breast to achieve rates of local control approaching 100%, is clear evidence that the disease burden is not the only factor determining local control. Evidence that margins, more widely clear than tumor not touching ink, decrease local recurrence in patients receiving whole breast RT is lacking, and the underlying biology of the tumor and the availability of targeted therapy appear to be the major determinants of local control. In recognition of the many factors impacting upon local control, a consensus conference concluded that the only negative margin width that could be endorsed for all patients with invasive carcinomas was tumor not touching ink.[59] This does not mean that in some circumstances a more widely clear margin is not appropriate; however, it does mean that the routine use of large surgical resection or mandatory re-excisions to obtain a more widely clear margin in all patients should be abandoned.

## 5.3 Margin Width and Local Recurrence: DCIS

All of the caveats regarding the lack of a standardized approach to margin assessment apply to DCIS as well as invasive cancer. In addition, because DCIS is not clinically detectable in the overwhelming majority of cases, limited sampling of margin specimens is particularly likely to underestimate the extent of DCIS. Three of the 4 randomized trials evaluating the benefit of RT in DCIS used a margin definition of tumor not touching ink,[60–62] while 20% patients in the SweDCIS study[63] had positive or unknown margins. Just as in the case of invasive cancer, level 1 evidence from randomized trials on the effect of increasing margin width on local recurrence is lacking. Low rates of local recurrence are seen with long-term follow-up in studies using the tumor not touching ink definition of a negative margin.

In spite of the lack of a boost dose of RT in NSABP B17,[61] the incidence of in-breast recurrence at a median follow-up of 17.3 years was 20%. In NSABP B24, this was reduced to 13.2% with the addition of tamoxifen, even though positive margins were allowed in this study.[61] In the United Kingdom–Australia–New Zealand DCIS study (UK–ANZ), after a median follow-up of 12.7 years, the incidence of in-breast recurrences was 10%.[62]

Dunne *et al.* performed a meta-analysis of 4,600 patients treated with BCT to examine the question of margin width. Patients with negative margins were significantly less likely than those with positive margins to experience local recurrence (OR, 0.36; 95% CI, 0.27%–0.47%). When specific margin widths were examined, patients with margins of 1 mm or less had a higher rate of local recurrence than those with more widely clear margins, but once a margin of 2 mm was obtained, no benefit for a more widely clear margin was seen (Table 5.3).[64] Of note, local recurrence was infrequent in all of the negative margin groups. In a study of 994 women with DCIS treated between 1985 and 2000, and identified through tumor registries in Monroe County, New York and the Henry Ford Health System, Detroit, Michigan, the multivariate relative risk of ipsilateral event-free survival for patients with margins less than 2 mm was 1.39 (95% CI, 0.71–2.73) compared to those with more widely clear margins.[65] This translates to an absolute difference of 1.6% at 5 years (95.6% versus 94.0%) and 3.2% at 10 years (90.5% versus 87.3%).

As previously discussed, DCIS may grow discontinuously in the ducts. In a study of 60 mastectomy specimens with DCIS, Faverly *et al.*[40] demonstrated that 50% had a discontinuous growth pattern. This was seen in only 10% of high-grade DCIS lesions compared to 70% of well-differentiated lesions and 55% of intermediate-grade lesions. These findings suggest that margins more widely clear than tumor not touching ink are particularly relevant for patients with low- and intermediate-grade DCIS. The presence of residual calcifications at the lumpectomy site is a powerful predictor of the presence of residual DCIS, and even when margins are negative, residual suspicious calcifications are an indication for re-excision.[66,67] Thus, margin

Table 5.3. Impact of margin width on local recurrence in DCIS.

| Negative margin width | Number | % In-breast recurrence | OR (95% CI) |
|---|---|---|---|
| Tumor not touching ink | 914 | 9.4 | 2.6 (1.1–7.3) |
| 1 mm | 1239 | 10.4 | 2.9 (1.3–8.1) |
| 2 mm | 207 | 5.8 | 1.5 (0.5–5.0) |
| ≥5 mm | 154 | 3.9 | 1.0 |

CI, confidence interval; DCIS, ductal carcinoma *in situ*; OR, odds ratio.
*Notes*: Data from Dunne *et al.*[64]

width and the findings of postexcision mammography are complimentary methods of assessing the completeness of an excision. As in the case of invasive cancer, the extent of DCIS approaching the margin and which margin is approached by DCIS warrant consideration as well.

A great deal of confusion regarding appropriate margin width in DCIS seems to have been engendered by the report of Silverstein *et al.*[68] that any DCIS lesion, regardless of size or grade that could be excised with a margin of 1 cm in all directions, did not require RT or tamoxifen. Many extrapolated these findings to indicate the need for a margin of 1 cm even when RT is used — an issue not addressed by Silverstein *et al.* The efforts to duplicate these findings in a multi-institutional setting have been unsuccessful to date. In the single-arm multi-institutional Intergroup CE 5194 study examining the role of excision alone in DCIS, margins of at least 3 mm and a negative postexcision mammogram were required. Patients with low- or intermediate-grade DCIS 2.5 cm or smaller in size and high-grade DCIS <1 cm in size were eligible. Approximately 50% of patients had negative margins of 1 cm or more. The 7-year rate of in-breast recurrence was 10.5% for the low- and intermediate-grade group compared with 19.0% for the high-grade group, but no significant impact of margins greater or less than 1 cm was noted for high-grade or non-high–grade lesions.[69] Thus, it is not even clear that margins of 1 cm or more are important when DCIS is treated with excision alone.

### 5.3.1 *DCIS: Summary and Conclusions*

The best available evidence, although somewhat limited, suggests that a margin of 2 mm in DCIS, coupled with a negative postexcision mammogram for calcification cases, reduces the risk of local recurrence compared to smaller negative margin widths. However, caution should be exercised before subjecting a patient to mastectomy or nipple removal to obtain an arbitrary predetermined margin width. As with invasive cancer, the extent of DCIS and other factors which impact upon the risk of local recurrence, such as patient age and willingness to take tamoxifen, are important in the decision-making process.

## References

1. Fisher B, Anderson S, Bryant J, *et al.* (2002) Twenty-year follow-up of a randomized trial comparing total mastectomy, lumpectomy, and lumpectomy plus irradiation following for the treatment of invasive breast cancer. *N Engl J Med* 347(16):1233–1241.

2. Veronesi U, Cascinelli N, Mariani L, *et al.* (2002) Twenty-year follow-up of a randomized study comparing breast-conserving surgery with radical mastectomy for early breast cancer. *N Engl J Med* 347(16):1227–1232.
3. Anderson SJ, Wapnir I, Dignam JJ, *et al.* (2009) Prognosis after ipsilateral breast tumor recurrence and locoregional recurrences in patients treated by breast-conserving therapy in five National Surgical Adjuvant Breast and Bowel Project protocols of node-negative breast cancer. *J Clin Oncol* 27(15):2466–2473.
4. Wapnir IL, Anderson SJ, Mamounas EP, *et al.* (2006) Prognosis after ipsilateral breast tumor recurrence and locoregional recurrences in five National Surgical Adjuvant Breast and Bowel Project node-positive adjuvant breast cancer trials. *J Clin Oncol* 24(13):2028–2037.
5. Morrow M, Jagsi R, Alderman AK, *et al.* (2009) Surgeon recommendations and receipt of mastectomy for treatment of breast cancer. *JAMA* 302(14):1551–1556.
6. Clarke M, Collins R, Darby S, *et al.* (2005) Effects of radiotherapy and of differences in the extent of surgery for early breast cancer on local recurrence and 15-year survival: An overview of the randomised trials. *Lancet* 366(9503):2087–2106.
7. Apple SK. (2006) Variability in gross and microscopic pathology reporting in excisional biopsies of breast cancer tissue. *Breast J* 12(2):145–149.
8. Molina MA, Snell S, Franceschi D, *et al.* (2009) Breast specimen orientation. *Ann Surg Oncol* 16(2):285–288.
9. Carter D. (1986) Margins of "lumpectomy" for breast cancer. *Hum Pathol* 17(4):330–332.
10. Guidi AJ, Connolly JL, Harris JR, Schnitt SJ. (1997) The relationship between shaved margin and inked margin status in breast excision specimens. *Cancer* 79(8):1568–1573.
11. Wright MJ, Park J, Fey JV, *et al.* (2007) Perpendicular inked versus tangential shaved margins in breast-conserving surgery: Does the method matter? *J Am Coll Surg* 204(4):541–549.
12. Huston TL, Pigalarga R, Osborne MP, Tousimis E. (2006) The influence of additional surgical margins on the total specimen volume excised and the reoperative rate after breast-conserving surgery. *Am J Surg* 192(4):509–512.
13. Jacobson AF, Asad J, Boolbol SK, *et al.* (2008) Do additional shaved margins at the time of lumpectomy eliminate the need for re-excision? *Am J Surg* 196(4):556–558.
14. Kobbermann A, Unzeitig A, Xie XJ, *et al.* (2011) Impact of routine cavity shave margins on breast cancer re-excision rates. *Ann Surg Oncol* 18(5):1349–1355.
15. Marudanayagam R, Singhal R, Tanchel B, *et al.* (2008) Effect of cavity shaving on reoperation rate following breast-conserving surgery. *Breast J* 14(6):570–573.
16. Rizzo M, Iyengar R, Gabram SG, *et al.* (2010) The effects of additional tumor cavity sampling at the time of breast-conserving surgery on final margin status, volume of resection, and pathologist workload. *Ann Surg Oncol* 17(1):228–234.

17. Tengher-Barna I, Hequet D, Reboul-Marty J, *et al.* (2009) Prevalence and predictive factors for the detection of carcinoma in cavity margin performed at the time of breast lumpectomy. *Mod Pathol* 22(2):299–305.
18. Cao D, Lin C, Woo SH, *et al.* (2005) Separate cavity margin sampling at the time of initial breast lumpectomy significantly reduces the need for reexcisions. *Am J Surg Pathol* 29(12):1625–1632.
19. Graham RA, Homer MJ, Katz J, *et al.* (2002) The pancake phenomenon contributes to the inaccuracy of margin assessment in patients with breast cancer. *Am J Surg* 184(2):89–93.
20. Azu M, Abrahamse P, Katz SJ, Jagsi R, Morrow M. (2010) What is an adequate margin for breast-conserving surgery? Surgeon attitudes and correlates. *Ann Surg Oncol* 17(2):558–563.
21. Taghian A, Mohiuddin M, Jagsi R, *et al.* (2005) Current perceptions regarding surgical margin status after breast-conserving therapy: Results of a survey. *Ann Surg* 241(4):629–639.
22. Waljee JF, Hu ES, Newman LA, Alderman AK. (2008) Predictors of re-excision among women undergoing breast-conserving surgery for cancer. *Ann Surg Oncol* 15(5):1297–1303.
23. Kurniawan ED, Wong MH, Windle I, *et al.* (2008) Predictors of surgical margin status in breast-conserving surgery within a breast screening program. *Ann Surg Oncol* 15(9):2542–2449.
24. Lovrics PJ, Cornacchi SD, Farrokhyar F, *et al.* (2010) Technical factors, surgeon case volume and positive margin rates after breast conservation surgery for early-stage breast cancer. *Can J Surg* 53(5):305–312.
25. Arriagada R, Le MG, Rochard F, Contesso G. (1996) Conservative treatment versus mastectomy in early breast cancer: Patterns of failure with 15 years of follow-up data. Institut Gustave-Roussy Breast Cancer Group. *J Clin Oncol* 14(5):1558–1564.
26. Blichert-Toft M, Rose C, Andersen JA, *et al.* (1992) Danish randomized trial comparing breast conservation therapy with mastectomy: Six years of life-table analysis. Danish Breast Cancer Cooperative Group. *J Natl Cancer Inst Monogr* (11):19–25.
27. Poggi MM, Danforth DN, Sciuto LC, *et al.* (2003) Eighteen-year results in the treatment of early breast carcinoma with mastectomy versus breast conservation therapy: The National Cancer Institute Randomized Trial. *Cancer* 98(4):697–702.
28. van Dongen JA, Voogd AC, Fentiman IS, *et al.* (2000) Long-term results of a randomized trial comparing breast-conserving therapy with mastectomy: European Organization for Research and Treatment of Cancer 10801 trial. *J Natl Cancer Inst* 92(14):1143–1150.
29. Veronesi U, Volterrani F, Luini A, *et al.* (1990) Quadrantectomy versus lumpectomy for small size breast cancer. *Eur J Cancer* 26(6):671–673.
30. Houssami N, Macaskill P, Marinovich ML, *et al.* (2010) Meta-analysis of the impact of surgical margins on local recurrence in women with early-stage invasive breast cancer treated with breast-conserving therapy. *Eur J Cancer* 46(18):3219–3232.

31. Dillon DA, Guidi AJ, Schnitt SJ. (2010) Pathology of invasive breast cancer. In: Harris JR, Lippman ME, Morrow M, Osborne CK (eds.), *Diseases of the Breast* 4th edn., Wolters Kluwer, Philadelphia, pp. 374–407.
32. Molland JG, Donnellan M, Janu NC, *et al.* (2004) Infiltrating lobular carcinoma — A comparison of diagnosis, management and outcome with infiltrating duct carcinoma. *Breast* 13(5):389–396.
33. Peiro G, Bornstein BA, Connolly JL, *et al.* (2000) The influence of infiltrating lobular carcinoma on the outcome of patients treated with breast-conserving surgery and radiation therapy. *Breast Cancer Res Treat* 59(1):49–54.
34. Santiago RJ, Harris EE, Qin L, *et al.* (2005) Similar long-term results of breast-conservation treatment for Stage I and II invasive lobular carcinoma compared with invasive ductal carcinoma of the breast: The University of Pennsylvania experience. *Cancer* 103(12):2447–2454.
35. Galimberti V, Maisonneuve P, Rotmensz N, *et al.* (2011) Influence of margin status on outcomes in lobular carcinoma: Experience of the European Institute of Oncology. *Ann Surg* 253(3):580–584.
36. Harris JR. (1996) Breast-conserving therapy as a model for creating new knowledge in clinical oncology. *Int J Radiat Oncol Biol Phys* 35(4):641–648.
37. Holland R, Connolly JL, Gelman R, *et al.* (1990) The presence of an extensive intraductal component following a limited excision correlates with prominent residual disease in the remainder of the breast. *J Clin Oncol* 8(1):113–118.
38. Bartelink H, Horiot JC, Poortmans P, *et al.* (2001) Recurrence rates after treatment of breast cancer with standard radiotherapy with or without additional radiation. *N Engl J Med* 345(19):1378–1387.
39. Park CC, Mitsumori M, Nixon A, *et al.* (2000) Outcome at 8 years after breast-conserving surgery and radiation therapy for invasive breast cancer: Influence of margin status and systemic therapy on local recurrence. *J Clin Oncol* 18(8):1668–1675.
40. Faverly DR, Burgers L, Bult P, Holland R. (1994) Three dimensional imaging of mammary ductal carcinoma *in situ*: Clinical implications. *Semin Diagn Pathol* 11(3):193–198.
41. Darvishian F, Hajdu SI, DeRisi DC. (2003) Significance of linear extent of breast carcinoma at surgical margin. *Ann Surg Oncol* 10(1):48–51.
42. Holland R, Veling SH, Mravunac M, Hendriks JH. (1985) Histologic multifocality of Tis, T1-2 breast carcinomas. Implications for clinical trials of breast-conserving surgery. *Cancer* 56(5):979–990.
43. Bartelink H, Horiot JC, Poortmans PM, *et al.* (2007) Impact of a higher radiation dose on local control and survival in breast-conserving therapy of early breast cancer: 10-year results of the randomized boost versus no boost EORTC 22881-10882 trial. *J Clin Oncol* 25(22):3259–3265.
44. Fisher B, Dignam J, Bryant J, *et al.* (1996) Five versus more than five years of tamoxifen therapy for breast cancer patients with negative lymph nodes and estrogen receptor-positive tumors. *J Natl Cancer Inst* 88(21):1529–1542.
45. Fisher B, Dignam J, Mamounas EP, *et al.* (1996) Sequential methotrexate and fluorouracil for the treatment of node-negative breast cancer patients with estrogen receptor-negative tumors: Eight-year results from National

Surgical Adjuvant Breast and Bowel Project (NSABP) B-13 and first report of findings from NSABP B-19 comparing methotrexate and fluorouracil with conventional cyclophosphamide, methotrexate, and fluorouracil. *J Clin Oncol* 14(7):1982–1992.

46. Romond EH, Perez EA, Bryant J, *et al.* (2005) Trastuzumab plus adjuvant chemotherapy for operable HER2-positive breast cancer. *N Engl J Med* 353(16):1673–1684.
47. Mamounas EP, Tang G, Fisher B, *et al.* (2010) Association between the 21-gene recurrence score assay and risk of locoregional recurrence in node-negative, estrogen receptor-positive breast cancer: Results from NSABP B-14 and NSABP B-20. *J Clin Oncol* 28(10):1677–1683.
48. Millar EK, Graham PH, O'Toole SA, *et al.* (2009) Prediction of local recurrence, distant metastases, and death after breast-conserving therapy in early-stage invasive breast cancer using a five-biomarker panel. *J Clin Oncol* 27(28):4701–4708.
49. Nguyen PL, Taghian AG, Katz MS, *et al.* (2008) Breast cancer subtype approximated by estrogen receptor, progesterone receptor, and HER-2 is associated with local and distant recurrence after breast-conserving therapy. *J Clin Oncol* 26(14):2373–2378.
50. Kyndi M, Sorensen FB, Knudsen H, *et al.* (2008) Estrogen receptor, progesterone receptor, HER-2, and response to postmastectomy radiotherapy in high-risk breast cancer: The Danish Breast Cancer Cooperative Group. *J Clin Oncol* 26(9):1419–1426.
51. Fisher B, Brown A, Mamounas E, *et al.* (1997) Effect of preoperative chemotherapy on local-regional disease in women with operable breast cancer: Findings from National Surgical Adjuvant Breast and Bowel Project B-18. *J Clin Oncol* 15(7):2483–2493.
52. van der Hage JA, van de Velde CJ, Julien JP, *et al.* (2001) Preoperative chemotherapy in primary operable breast cancer: Results from the European Organization for Research and Treatment of Cancer trial 10902. *J Clin Oncol* 19(22):4224–4237.
53. Mieog JS, van der Hage JA, van de Velde CJ. (2007) Preoperative chemotherapy for women with operable breast cancer. *Cochrane Database Syst Rev* (2):CD005002.
54. Wolmark N, Wang J, Mamounas E, *et al.* (2001) Preoperative chemotherapy in patients with operable breast cancer: Nine-year results from National Surgical Adjuvant Breast and Bowel Project B-18. *J Natl Cancer Inst Monogr* (30):96–102.
55. Hylton N. (2006) MR imaging for assessment of breast cancer response to neoadjuvant chemotherapy. *Magn Reson Imaging Clin N Am* 14(3): 383–389, vii.
56. Chen AM, Meric-Bernstam F, Hunt KK, *et al.* (2004) Breast conservation after neoadjuvant chemotherapy: The MD Anderson Cancer Center Experience. *J Clin Oncol* 22(12):2303–2312.
57. Meyers MO, Klauber-Demore N, Ollila DW, *et al.* (2011) Impact of breast cancer molecular subtypes on locoregional recurrence in patients treated

with neoadjuvant chemotherapy for locally advanced breast cancer. *Ann Surg Oncol* 18(10):2851–2857.
58. Morrow M, Harris JR. (2007) Practice guideline for breast conservation therapy in the management of invasive breast cancer. *J Am Coll Surg* 205:362–376.
59. Kaufmann M, Morrow M, von Minckwitz G, Harris JR. (2010) Locoregional treatment of primary breast cancer: Consensus recommendations from an International Expert Panel. *Cancer* 116(5):1184–1191.
60. Bijker N, Meijnen P, Peterse JL, *et al.* EORTC Breast Cancer Cooperative Group; EORTC Radiotherapy Group. (2006) Breast-conserving treatment with or without radiotherapy in ductal carcinoma-in-situ: Ten-year results of European Organisation for Research and Treatment of Cancer randomized phase III trial 10853 — A study by the EORTC Breast Cancer Cooperative Group and EORTC Radiotherapy Group. *J Clin Oncol* 24(21):3381–3387.
61. Wapnir IL, Dignam JJ, Fisher B, *et al.* (2011) Long-term outcomes of invasive ipsilateral breast tumor recurrences after lumpectomy in NSABP B-17 and B-24 randomized clinical trials for DCIS. *J Natl Cancer Inst* 103(6): 478–488.
62. Cuzick J, Sestak I, Pinder SE, *et al.* (2011) Effect of tamoxifen and radiotherapy in women with locally excised ductal carcinoma *in situ*: Long-term results from the UK/ANZ DCIS trial. *Lancet Oncol* 12(1):21–29.
63. Emdin SO, Granstrand B, Ringberg A, *et al.* (2006) SweDCIS: Radiotherapy after sector resection for ductal carcinoma *in situ* of the breast. Results of a randomised trial in a population offered mammography screening. *Acta Oncol* 45(5):536–543.
64. Dunne C, Burke JP, Morrow M, Kell MR. (2009) Effect of margin status on local recurrence after breast conservation and radiation therapy for ductal carcinoma *in situ*. J Clin Oncol 27(10):1615–1620.
65. Dick AW, Sorbero MS, Ahrendt GM, *et al.* (2011) Comparative effectiveness of ductal carcinoma *in situ* management and the roles of margins and surgeons. *J Natl Cancer Inst* 103(2):92–104.
66. Aref A, Youssef E,Washington T, *et al.* (2000) The value of postlumpectomy mammogram in the management of breast cancer patients presenting with suspicious microcalcifications. *Cancer J Sci Am* 6(1):25–27.
67. Gluck BS, Dershaw DD, Liberman L, Deutch BM. (1993) Microcalcifications on postoperative mammograms as an indicator of adequacy of tumor excision. *Radiology* 188(2):469–472.
68. Silverstein MJ, Lagios MD, Groshen S, *et al.* (1999) The influence of margin width on local control of ductal carcinoma *in situ* of the breast. *N Engl J Med* 340(19):1455–1461.
69. Hughes LL, Wang M, Page DL, *et al.* (2009) Local excision alone without irradiation for ductal carcinoma *in situ* of the breast: A trial of the Eastern Cooperative Oncology Group. *J Clin Oncol* 27(32):5319–5324.

# Chapter 6

# RESECTION OF THE TUMOR

Mahmoud El-Tamer
*Breast Service, Department of Surgery,*
*Memorial Sloan-Kettering Cancer Center,*
*New York, NY 10065, USA*

## 6.1 General Principles and Preoperative Planning

The preliminary objective of an oncoplastic surgical procedure must always be adequate resection of the primary tumor. The surgeon should not compromise that objective. An adequate resection is defined as the complete removal of the tumor with histologically confirmed negative margins. We have defined in Chapter 5 what we consider to be evidence-based negative margins. Surgeons should follow these recommendations or resort to their departmental or institutional definitions as long as histologically negative margins are achieved.

Positive margins, however defined, have been associated with a significantly higher incidence of recurrence.[1,2] Furthermore, some have reported an association between positive margins, and systemic recurrence and disease-specific survival.[3] All efforts should be directed toward achieving negative margins from the start, particularly when complex repairs are planned, or when breast reduction or rotation flaps are used. The aim of the oncoplastic resection is to maximize the removal of malignant tissue and minimize the loss of benign tissue, including skin, subcutaneous fat, breast, pectoralis fascia, and muscle tissue. We recommend excising extra benign tissue for the purpose of breast reduction or mastopexy only when indicated.

One of the most important steps in managing a breast cancer is achieving a diagnosis prior to any surgical intervention. Percutaneous needle aspiration or biopsy is currently the standard of care. Preoperative diagnosis by needle biopsy can be achieved in more than 90% of patients.[4] Preoperative needle diagnosis limits the number of operative procedures[5] and increases the sentinel node detection rate.[6]

Preoperative evaluation of the size and extent of the tumor is crucial for planning the resection. All available images are reviewed and should be accessible to the surgeons during the operative procedure as needed. Mammography, ultrasonography, and magnetic resonance imaging (MRI) are complementary when defining the extent of the disease. Mammography has the unique capability of defining the extent of malignant and suspicious calcifications. When the calcifications are at a distance from the index cancer or may not be included in the planned resection, we have felt it more convenient to use a separate needle or wire for localization, even when the primary is palpable. As mammograms are performed in the standing position and under breast compression, of particular concern is that the calcification may not be in the expected location when the patient is lying down on the operative table. Mammography and ultrasonography in particular are helpful in defining the size of the malignant mass.

The role of MRI in evaluating the extent of disease has been heavily debated over the past few years. MRI has been helpful but occasionally deceptive in planning resection. MRI has not decreased the re-excision rate and certainly has not lowered the rate of local recurrence.[7] Furthermore, some clinicians have reported an unnecessary mastectomy rate in 5% to 10% of cases when using MRI for evaluation of the extent of disease. So far, we have not uniformly relied on MRI to evaluate the extent of disease. We have limited MRI to patients who fall into the following categories:

(1) Mammographically occult lesions.
(2) Premenopausal women with dense breasts, particularly women younger than 40 years of age.
(3) Patients considering contralateral prophylactic mastectomy.
(4) High-risk patients, particularly those who are mutation carriers.

The patient is marked preoperatively in the pre-anesthesia care unit. We prefer to mark the patient while she is standing or in a semi-sitting position. In patients for whom a major resection is contemplated with mobilization of the nipple areola complex (NAC), certain landmarks should be defined and marked preoperatively as described in Chapter 2. We strongly encourage the breast/general surgeon who has not had any training in mastopexy or breast reduction to seek the expertise of a plastic surgeon. In cases where the resection is limited and will not involve any mobilization of the NAC of the breast, the skin incision may be drawn intraoperatively while the patient is on the table. We do, however, feel that the lines of Kraissl[7,8] are better defined in the standing position. The areolar edges in fair individuals or nulliparous women are better visualized before prepping the patient, particularly when using Betadine as a surgical preparation.

The vast majority of breast conservation procedures are performed under local anesthesia with sedation. In cases where we have planned a major resection with repositioning of the NAC, particularly when a breast reduction or a mastopexy procedure is included, we have resorted to general anesthesia.

## 6.2 Resection of the Primary

### 6.2.1 *General Principles*

Breast surgery has long been dominated by Halstedian principles. With the paradigm shift from mastectomy to breast conservation, some surgeons have applied the same Halstedian principles to the local excision of the breast primary; such an approach recommends an *en bloc* resection starting with the overlying skin, the breast cancer with the breast tissue surrounding it, and down to the chest muscles, including the pectoralis fascia. Such a composite resection was the main approach utilized in the Milan breast-conserving therapy trial and was labeled "quadrantectomy." The National Surgical Adjuvant Breast and Bowel Project (NSABP) trial recommended a lumpectomy in the form of a wide-local excision without necessarily including the overlying skin and underlying pectoralis fascia in every resection. This approach was labeled as lumpectomy. Both studies have shown the reliability of breast-conservation surgery when compared with mastectomy with 20 years follow-up. Both trials also demonstrated a similar rate of local recurrence of the original primary when compared with mastectomy. The incidence of local recurrence in the NSABP trial was higher than the Milan trial. The inclusion criteria were different, however; the Milan trial was limited to T1 tumors whereas the NSABP included lesions as large as 5 cm in size. Although intuitive, there are enough data to support that larger resections will result in more deformity without improving local control. Noh *et al.* compared 456 patients who underwent a quadrantectomy with 351 patients whose surgical procedures were limited to a lumpectomy. Both groups had similar clinical and pathologic characteristics. Using multivariate analysis, young age (less than 35 years), positive nodes, and the presence of an extensive intraductal component were the only predictors of local recurrence. Lumpectomy was not a predictor of local recurrence; however, it was associated with a higher re-excision rate. The conclusion was that the extent of surgery did not predict ipsilateral breast tumor recurrence when adequate surgical margins were achieved.[9]

To avoid a high re-excision rate, we have removed the primary tumor and excised separate margins. We have focused our surgical resection on the tumor and appropriate clear margins. We have limited excision of the overlying skin or underlying pectoralis fascia to tumors that are close to these structures. Frequently, however, we recommend excision of the overlying skin to facilitate approximation of breast tissue and avoid redundant skin, or as part of a mastopexy or breast reduction procedure.

### 6.2.2 *Technical Aspects*

Following completion of the incision, we elevate the skin and subcutaneous tissue off the underlying breast. We use the superficial fascial plane as if we were performing a mastectomy [Figure 6.1(a)] when the tumor is quite superficial. If the tumor is deep in the breast tissue, we believe the surgeon can save a significant amount of tissue and raise the flaps at the glandular level [Figure 6.1(b)] or even deeper in the breast, particularly in centrally located and deep tumors. One caveat, however: when one raises the flaps in the breast substance, attention must be directed to the anterior margins in the specimen. We prefer to excise the overlying skin if we feel we must include the subcutaneous tissue in the resection to achieve a sound oncologic procedure. We have noticed that resection of the subcutaneous tissue from the dermis down has routinely resulted in a poor cosmetic outcome, with the dermis adhering to the underlying tissue, resulting in a retracted scar. The flap elevation prior to resection allows for excellent visualization and planning of breast tissue resection [Figure 6.1(c)].

We have recently adopted a technique in which we excise the tumor with 0.5–1.0 cm grossly negative margins. After completion of this limited lumpectomy, we re-excise the totality of the lumpectomy cavity and submit each edge of the lumpectomy cavity separately as final margins while orienting the new true margin for the pathologist. We, as well as others, have recognized a drop in our re-excision rate as a result. Our resection has been dictated by the location of the tumor and has not compromised the final cosmetic result. When we combine resection of a tumor with a breast reduction (see Chapter 8), we usually resect the whole quadrant where the tumor is located with 2–3 cm grossly negative margins as part of the reductive procedure.

Some surgeons have advocated the use of intraoperative ultrasound (US) for guidance.[10,11] It is certainly a useful tool as described in the literature and reported by others. We have not routinely used intraoperative

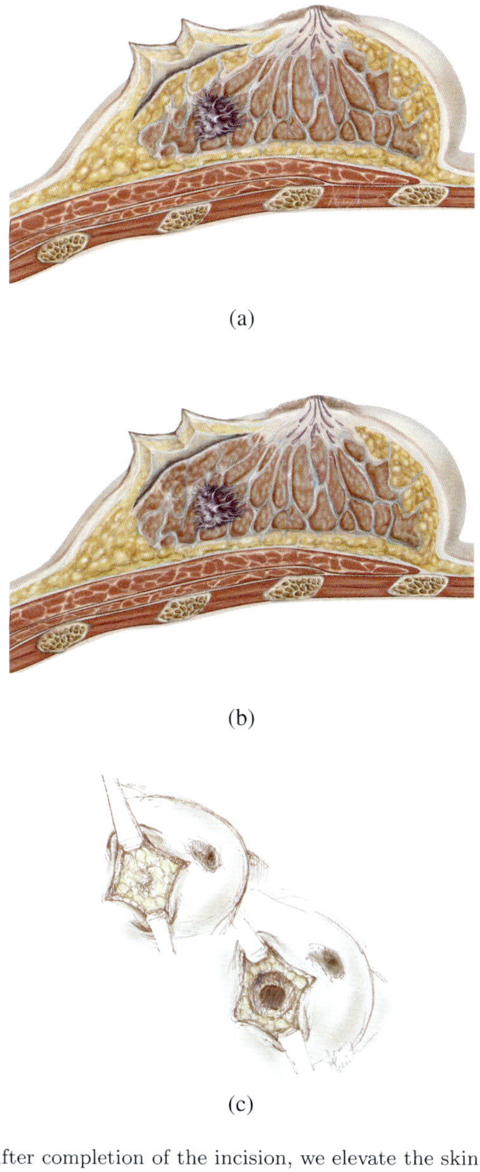

(a)

(b)

(c)

Figure 6.1. (a) After completion of the incision, we elevate the skin and subcutaneous tissue off the underlying breast following the superficial fascial plane as if we were performing a mastectomy. (b) If the tumor is deep in the breast tissue, we believe surgeons can spare a significant amount of tissue and raise the flaps at the glandular level. (c) Flap elevation prior to resection allows for excellent visualization and planning of the breast tissue to be excised.

US for guidance while excising tumors. With our lumpectomy technique, positive margins are most frequently due to ductal carcinoma *in situ* (DCIS) where ultrasound has a limited role. However, we have used needle localization liberally in patients in whom the tumor is vaguely palpable. We have also asked radiologists to aim for the center of the tumor while localizing a lesion. We have preferred the bracketing technique to a single needle in the center of the microcalcifications when dealing with a wide area of microcalcifications. The bracketing technique can help to better identify the limits of the resection, particularly when the calcifications are spread more than 3 cm in width (see Case No. 1).

Case No. 1

A 60-year-old patient presented with a new mammographic finding of 7.5-cm microcalcifications. She was interested in BCT. The bracketing technique was used to delineate the extent of resection in the left breast.

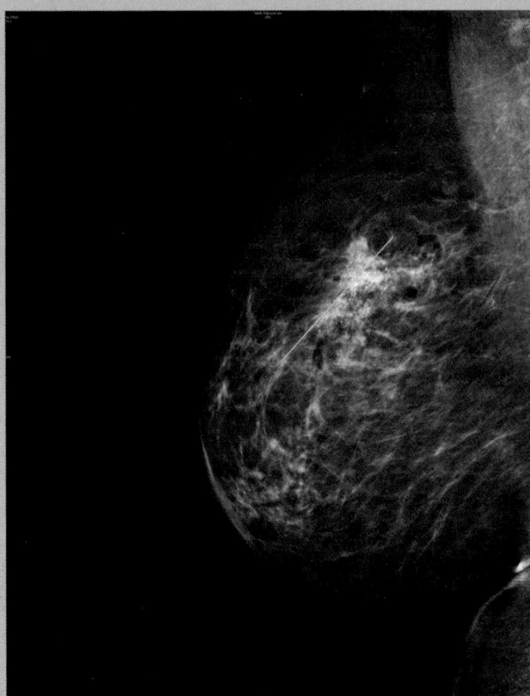

Image 1.1. Left breast medio-lateral oblique.

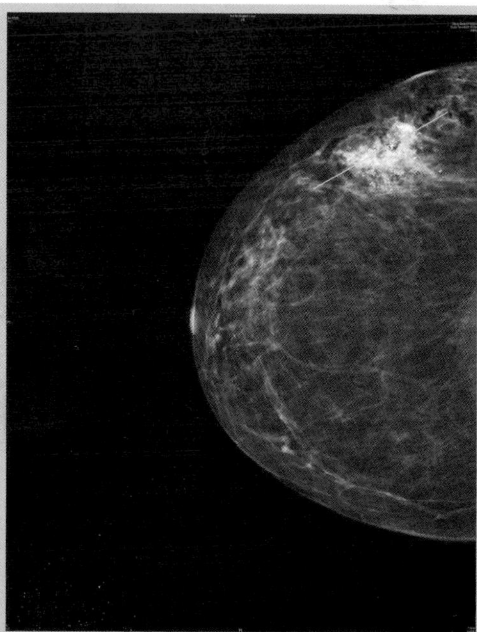

Image 1.2. Left breast cranio-caudal.

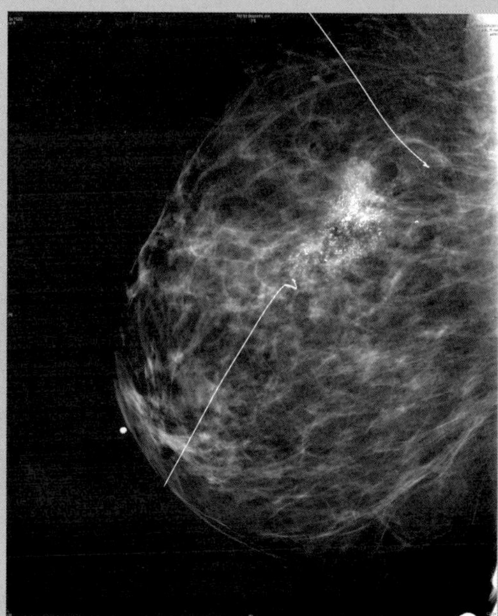

Image 1.3. Left breast preoperative needle localization with bracketing.

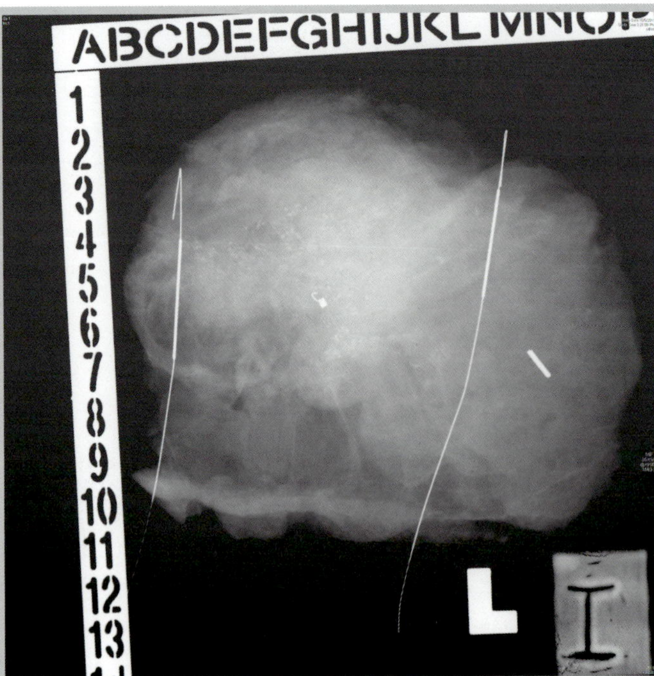


Image 1.4. Specimen X-ray. The lumpectomy measured 11 cm × 10 cm × 6 cm.

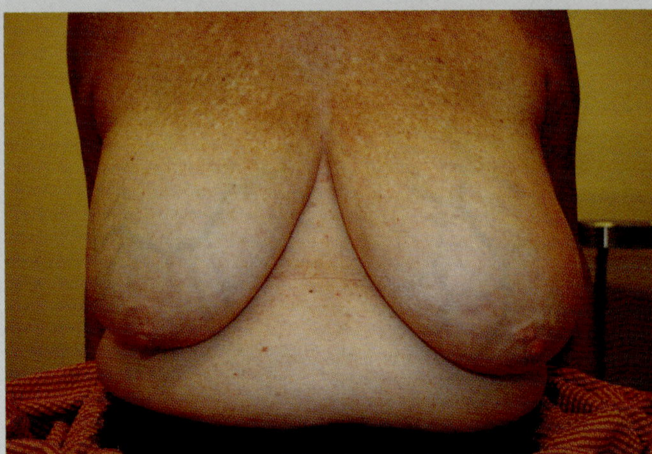

Image 1.5. The patient after left breast lumpectomy and sentinel node biopsy.

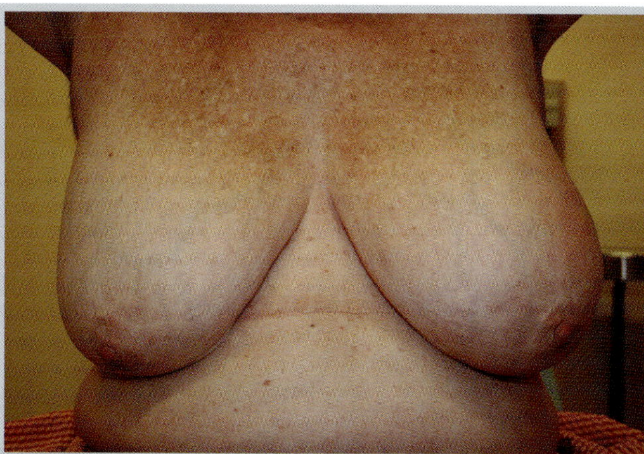

Image 1.6. The patient after left breast lumpectomy and sentinel node biopsy with the arm elevated. Notice the minimal deformity.

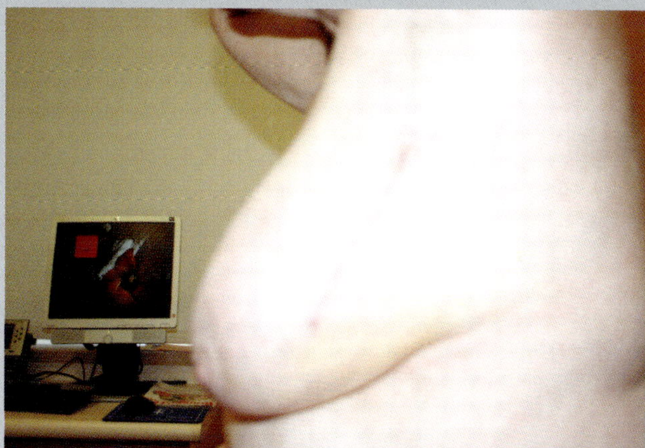

Image 1.7. The lateral view showing the scar.

Prior to adopting the technique of excising and submitting the margins separately, we used to perform a lumpectomy with 1–2 cm grossly negative margins. Whatever technique the surgeon uses, we strongly recommend orienting the specimen intraoperatively. Different methods have been used to orient the specimen, including sutures, hemoclips, and metallic markers. Some surgeons have even resorted to inking the specimen intraoperatively. We believe each breast center should develop and adhere to a convenient method of specimen orientation that is agreed upon by pathologists and surgeons. With clearly defined margins, we have limited re-excision to the positive margins only. We have reserved whole cavity re-excision to multifocal disease with multiple positive margins, or to cases referred to us following lumpectomy with unoriented specimens. Gibson *et al.* did not notice any difference in local recurrence following ink-directed re-excision and whole cavity re-excision for positive margins. Specimen weights after whole cavity re-excision were nearly 4 times heavier than ink-directed limited re-excision (23 g versus 83 g). Larger volumes of tissue excision will clearly negatively impact the cosmetic outcome.[12]

After completion of removal of the primary, we repair the defect and close the overlying skin. (See Chapter 7 for the techniques of repair.) We do not usually insert drains into the breast tissue. In cases where we perform the resection and complete an axillary node dissection, we may consider inserting a drain into the breast tissue, particularly when the tumor is located in the outer quadrant or centrally. The surgical dressing we apply is limited to steri-strips and a transparent impermeable dressing such as an Opsite® or a Tegaderm®. We do not wrap patients with Ace bandages; we have routinely asked the patient to continuously wear a surgical or wireless sports brassiere continuously for a period of 72–96 hours, however.

In the postoperative period, patients are allowed to shower as of the first operative day and resume regular daily activity. We recommend that patients abstain from applying heavy pressure over the operated breast and refrain from physical activities that result in heavy bouncing of the breast (such as jogging and heavy cardiovascular exercises) for a period of 6 to 8 weeks. We avoid any mammographic studies in the postoperative period unless essential, and then we limit the amount of compression to the bare minimum for fear of disrupting the repair, particularly in women with fatty breasts. In cases where the patient is returning to the operating room for re-excision of margins, we repeat the mammogram as necessary prior to the re-excision to identify residual calcification.

In very few cases with significant disruption of the lymphatic drainage, we have encountered a significant seroma. The seroma, however, has not been significant enough to disrupt the repair. In our experience, the seroma resulted in disruption of the repair in only one patient, necessitating a return to the operating room for evacuation of seroma and re-approximation of tissue. Most seroma are adequately managed with percutaneous office aspiration as needed.

## References

1. Schnitt SJ. (2003) Risk factors for local recurrence in patients with invasive breast cancer and negative surgical margins of excision. Where are we and where are we going? *Am J Clin Pathol* 120(4):485–488.

2. Singletary SE. (2002) Surgical margins in patients with early-stage breast cancer treated with breast conservation therapy. *Am J Surg* 184(5):383–393.
3. Meric F, Mirza NQ, Vlastos G, *et al.* (2003) Positive surgical margins and ipsilateral breast tumor recurrence predict disease-specific survival after breast-conserving therapy. *Cancer* 97(4):926–933.
4. Pocock B, Taback B, Klein L, *et al.* (2009) Preoperative needle biopsy as a potential quality measure in breast cancer surgery. *Ann Surg Oncol* 16(5):1108–1111.
5. Morrow M, Venta L, Stinson T, Bennett C. (2001) Prospective comparison of stereotactic core biopsy and surgical excision as diagnostic procedures for breast cancer patients. *Ann Surg* 233(4):537–541.
6. Julian TB, Land SR, Fourchotte V, *et al.* (2007) Is sentinel node biopsy necessary in conservatively treated DCIS? *Ann Surg Oncol* 14(8):2202–2208.
7. Gray H. (1995) Skin lines. In: Williams PL (ed.), *Gray's Anatomy*, 38th edn. Churchil Livingstone, London, pp. 378–381.
8. Kraissl CJ. (1951) The selection of appropriate lines for elective surgical incisions. *Plast Reconstr Surg (1946)* 8(1):1–28.
9. Noh WC, Paik NS, Kim MS, *et al.* (2005) Ipsilateral breast tumor recurrence after breast-conserving therapy: A comparison of quadrantectomy versus lumpectomy at a single institution. *World J Surg* 29(8):1001–1006.
10. Buman SJ, Clark DA. (2005) Breast intraoperative ultrasound: Prospective study in 112 patients with impalpable lesions. *ANZ J Surg* 75(3):124–127.
11. Ngo C, Pollet AG, Laperrelle J, *et al.* (2007) Intraoperative ultrasound localization of nonpalpable breast cancers. *Ann Surg Oncol* 14(9):2485–2489.
12. Gibson GR, Lesnikoski BA, Yoo J, *et al.* (2001) A comparison of ink-directed and traditional whole-cavity re-excision for breast lumpectomy specimens with positive margins. *Ann Surg Oncol* 8(9):693–704.

# Chapter 7

# REPAIR OF BREAST DEFECTS

Mahmoud El-Tamer

*Breast Service, Department of Surgery,*
*Memorial Sloan-Kettering Cancer Center,*
*New York, NY 10065, USA*

The resection, as previously described in Chapter 6, is centered on the tumor. It has been our practice to excise the primary with 0.5–1.0 cm of grossly soft tissue and later excise each margin separately. We have noticed a decrease in our re-excision rate with perhaps a subtle increase in the volume of resection. With separate excision of margins, it was easier for the surgeon and the pathologist to clearly agree on the exact margin. We mark the site of the true margin intraoperatively. This mode of resection and orientation works well for us at Memorial Sloan-Kettering Cancer Center. We recommend, however, that you follow your institutional practice. We do not necessarily perform a full-thickness resection, that is, from skin down to the pectoralis fascia, on every patient. Following completion of the resection, we evaluate the mobility of the breast tissue.

When the breast tissue does not have enough mobility over the chest wall, we then elevate the breast tissue off the pectoralis fascia in the plane of the retromammary space.

The defect is evaluated for closure and is approximated along the most convenient route for the particular quadrant where it is located. The skin overlying the breast tissue is elevated when the tumor is close to the surface or when dealing with A or B cup size breasts. In deep-seated tumors, we resect the lesion, repair the defect, and later assess the need for further skin elevation.

The resection and repair of defect are planned based on multiple factors:

- The location of the tumor (quadrant and depth)
- The size of the tumor

- The size of the breast
- The level of ptosis of the breast

In patients for whom the resection would include less than 25% of the breast volume, a simple oncoplastic procedure can easily be performed. In cases in which the patient has a ptotic breast or is interested in reducing the size of her breast, we would encourage combining the oncologic procedure with a mastopexy or a breast reduction, accordingly.

## 7.1 General Principles

The skin incision is performed, and the skin and subcutaneous tissue are elevated off the breast for a distance of 2–4 cm circumferentially around the center of the tumor as indicated in Figure 7.1(a). When the tumor is very close to the skin or tethering the skin, we recommend excision of the overlying skin as part of the specimen. If the tumor is very close to the superficial layer of breast glandular tissue, we elevate the skin in the mastectomy plane [Figure 7.1(b)]. When the tumor is in the center of the gland, we elevate the skin at the glandular level [Figure 7.1(c)]. In cases where the tumor is deep in the center of the breast, we continue the dissection down in the breast tissue up to 1–2 cm above the tumor, and then start the resection at that level.

The lesion is excised as per your routine. At the beginning of this chapter, we have summarized our personal technique. We recommend orienting the specimen by whatever methods the surgeon or the institution deem appropriate. We cannot, however, overstress the importance of specimen orientation.

In A and B cup size breasts, we have invariably realized that the resection is full thickness, that is, down to the pectoralis major fascia, due to the paucity of breast tissue surrounding the tumor. In larger breasts, we have limited full-thickness resection depending on the location and size of the tumor. Following completion of the resection [Figure 7.1(d)], the sub-glandular space or retromammary bursa is entered. The mobility of the breast is assessed; the breast tissue is elevated off the pectoralis fascia using the retromammary plane. In some areas, and particularly in the center of the breast, there may be no need to undermine the breast tissue [Figure 7.1(e)]. The breast tissue is rotated or advanced as necessary, and it is approximated with sutures. We have routinely used absorbable sutures of 2-0 or 3-0 thickness. The type of rotation/advancement and approximation vary with the quadrant of the tumor. The main purpose of mobilizing the breast tissue is to allow the restoration of contour and closure of the defect. When the defect is left open, a seroma develops in the immediate

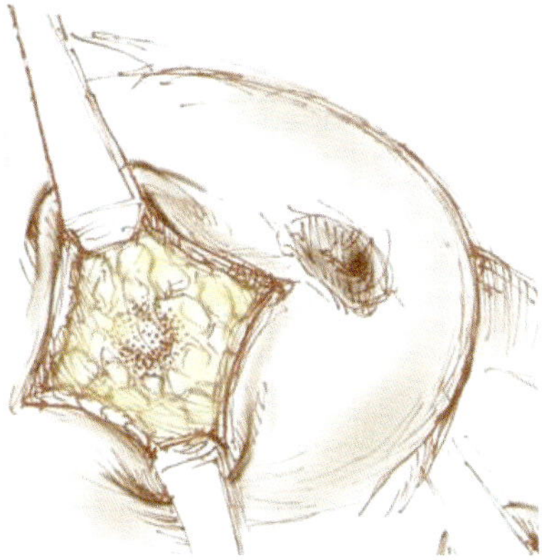

(a)

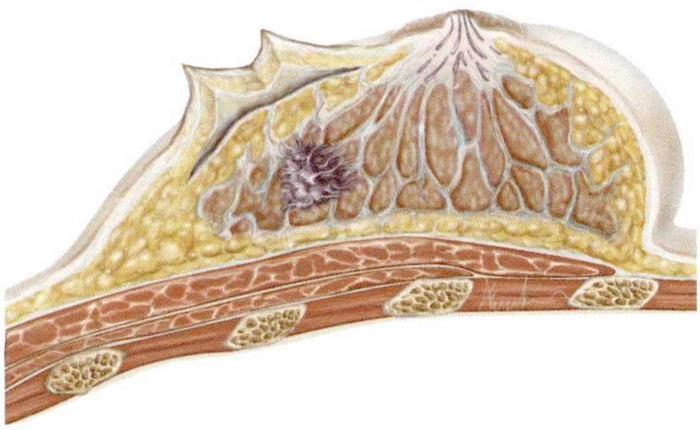

(b)

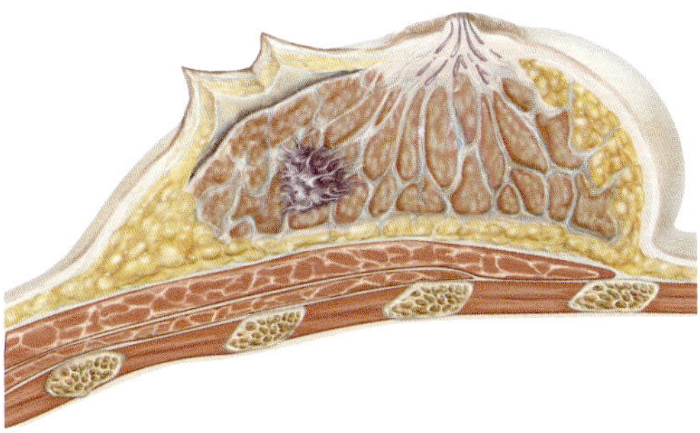

(c)

Figure 7.1. (a) Skin elevation prior to resection. (b) The plane of elevation is in the subcutaneous tissue as if performing a mastectomy. (c) The level of skin elevation is at the glandular level. The skin flap thickness varies with the amount of subcutaneous tissue. (d) This is a patient who underwent a resection of a lateral tumor. The resection extended from the skin down to the pectoralis muscle. (e) The breast tissue is shown after its separation from the pectoralis fascia in preparation for a radial closure.

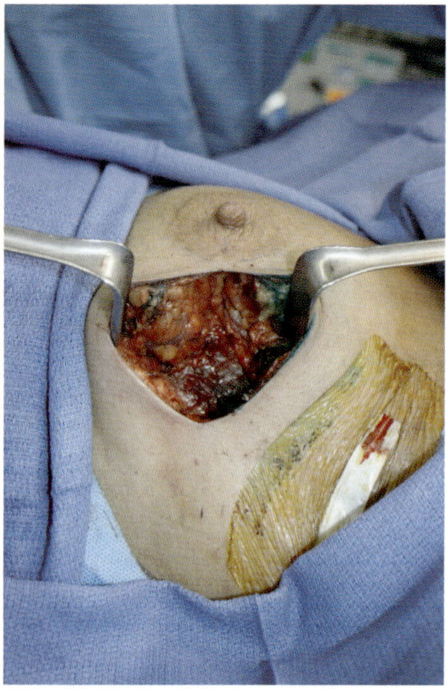

(d)

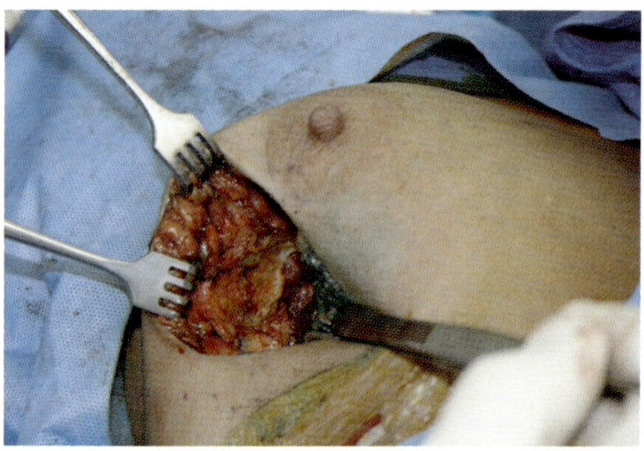

(e)

Figure 7.1. (*Continued*)

postoperative period, therefore giving fullness to the breast. With time, the seroma resolves and the patient receives radiation therapy, resulting in shrinkage of the cavity and some deformity of contour. Frequently, the skin will adhere to the underlying muscle, creating a significant deformity of the breast. Such deformities are particularly seen following resection of inner quadrant lesions. We have also observed that in patients for whom the lumpectomy cavity is not approximated, the resulting scar is larger and denser, making follow-up clinical exams and mammograms more difficult compared with cases in which the lumpectomy defect has been repaired.

In most women, there are some differences in the size and shape of both breasts. This asymmetry varies from the subtle to the grossly obvious.[1] It is quite understandable that following an oncologic procedure, there will be loss of volume and some differences in breast size and shape. One hopes, however, that with the plastic aspect of the oncoplastic procedure, this difference will be minimized. In spite of the size difference, the final shape of the operated breast will be cosmetically acceptable and frequently preferable to the contralateral side.

All the described techniques in this section are performed without specific attempts at mobilization of the nipple. In patients for whom the resection would require removal of more than 20%–25% of breast volume, we feel that such a resection needs to be part of a breast reduction, and we reserve such procedures to C cup size breasts or larger. We prefer to start patients with A and B cup size breasts who would require removal of more than 25%–30% of the breast on neoadjuvant therapy, if indicated, in an attempt to reduce the volume of resection to achieve better cosmetic results. Refer to Chapter 3 for neoadjuvant therapy.

We have generally used 5 types of closures that we will describe independently:

- Transverse closure
- Radial closure
- Triangular closure
- Purse-string closure
- Mobilization of surrounding subcutaneous tissue

### 7.1.1 *Transverse Closure*

Transverse closure is completed by advancing the upper and lower edges of the defect toward each other, resulting in a transverse line of closure [Figures 7.2(a)–(c)]. This type of closure is ideal for the defects located in the upper hemisphere and the center of the breast. We have avoided using this type of closure in the lower hemisphere, particularly for defects located between 4 o'clock and 8 o'clock, as it will invariably result in a downward traction of the nipple areola complex (NAC). To avoid such traction, one may have to elevate the NAC off the glandular flap.

Case Nos. 1 and 2 demonstrate the technique and the postoperative results *in vivo*. Case No. 3 shows the result of transverse closure in the upper inner quadrant.

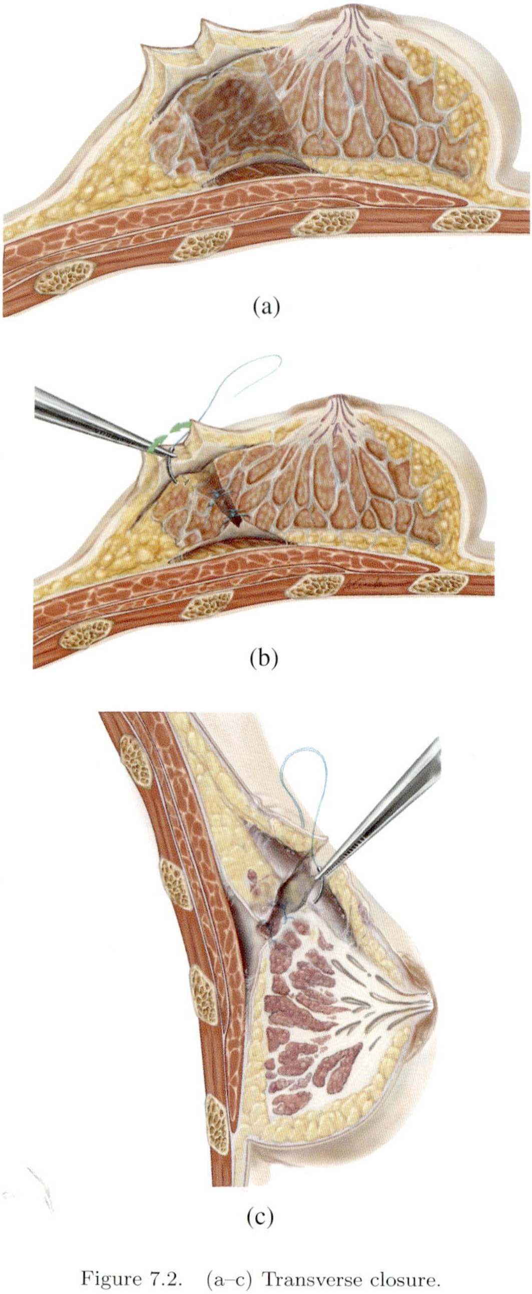

Figure 7.2. (a–c) Transverse closure.

Case Nos. 1 and 2: Patients with transverse closure at 12 o'clock.

Case No. 1

This patient presented with a 2.5-cm tumor in the 12 o'clock axis. She was scheduled for a needle localization lumpectomy and sentinel node biopsy.

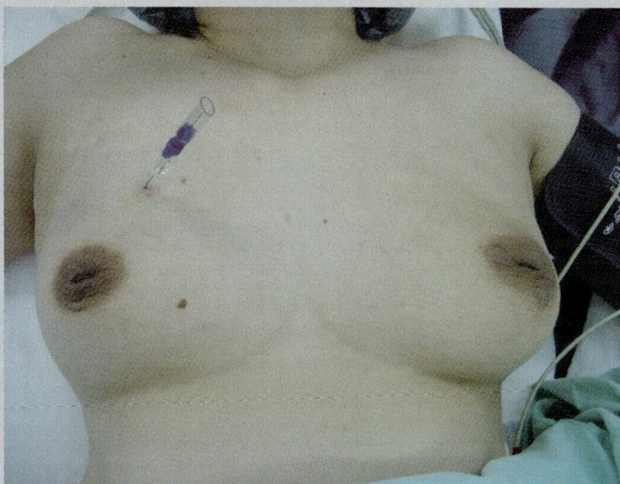

Image 1.1. The patient on the operating room table with needle localization.

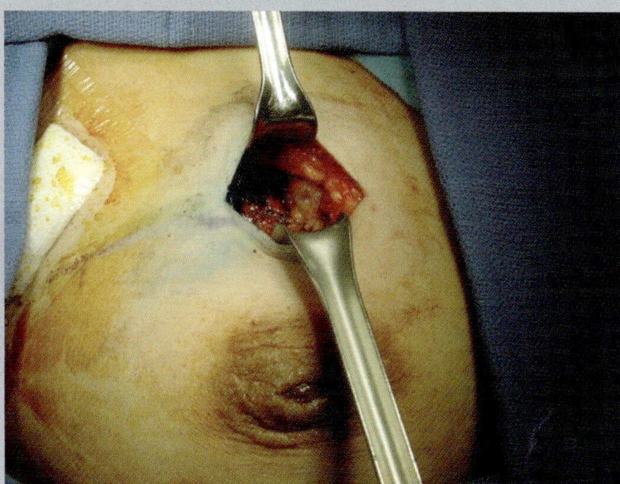

Image 1.2. The patient after completion of resection. The dressing in the axilla was applied over the sentinel node scar.

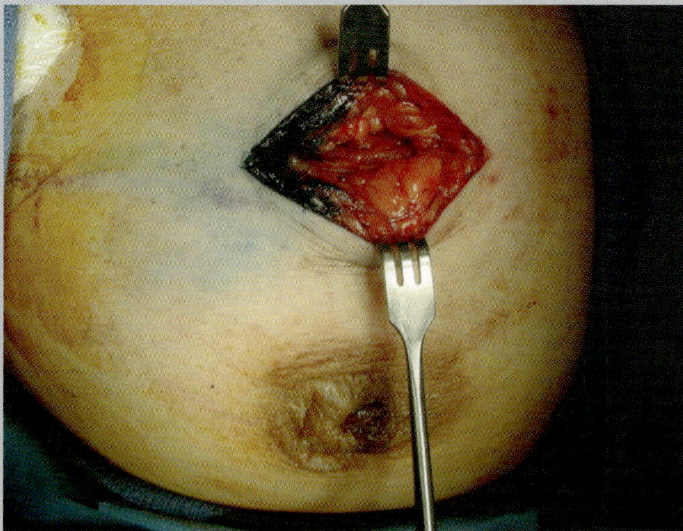

Image 1.3. The breast flaps elevated off the pectoralis fascia and overlying skin. The flaps are prepared for transverse approximation.

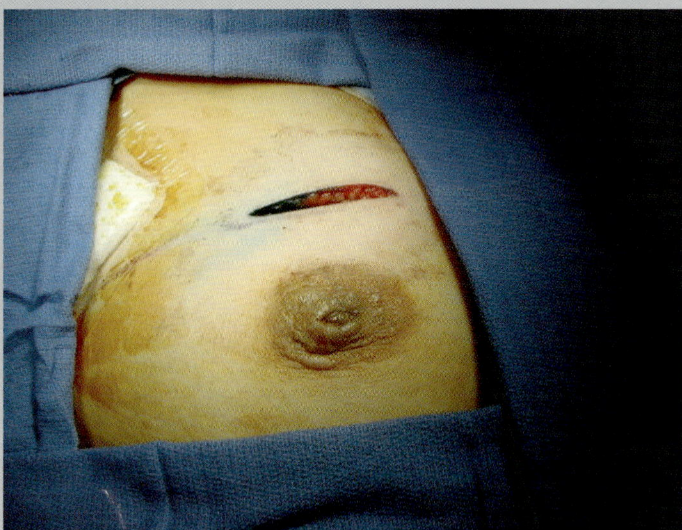

Image 1.4. The patient after completion of the breast tissue approximation, prior to closure of the skin.

Case No. 2. This patient with size A cup breasts had a 2.5-cm tumor in the same location as the patient in Case No. 1.

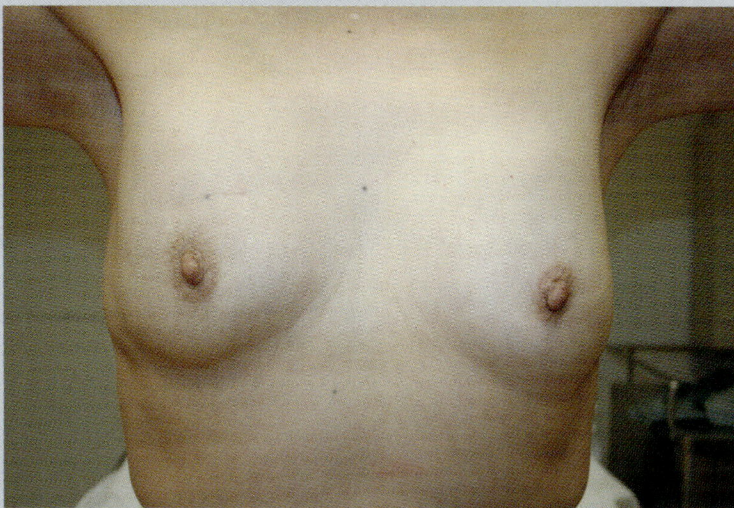

Image 2.1. This patient with similar size and location of tumor seen 7 years postoperatively. The patient reported that she preferred the operated breast because it "looked younger."

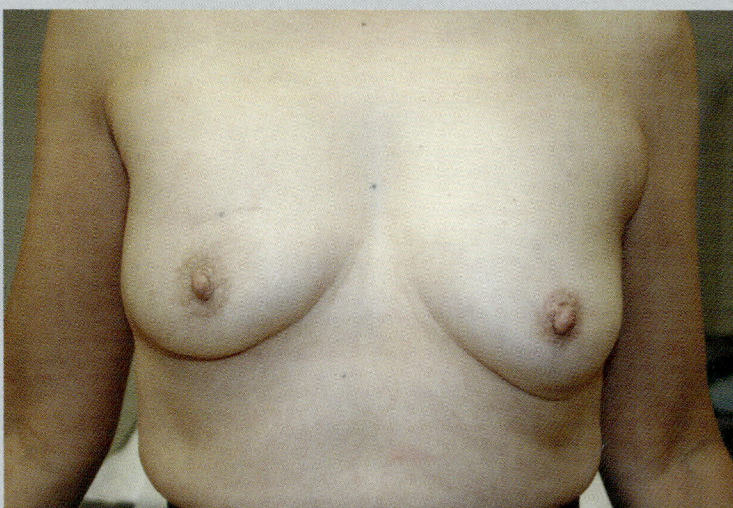

Image 2.2. Same patient as in Image 2.1.

Case No. 3: Transverse repair in the upper inner quadrant (UIQ).

- Images 3.1 and 3.2 show the patient 2 years after lumpectomy and sentinel node biopsy for a T2N0 tumor located in the UIQ. Notice the size difference of both breasts and the subtle elevation of the inframammary line with arm elevation. Except for that critical observation, the patient was very happy with the contour and shape of the operated breast.

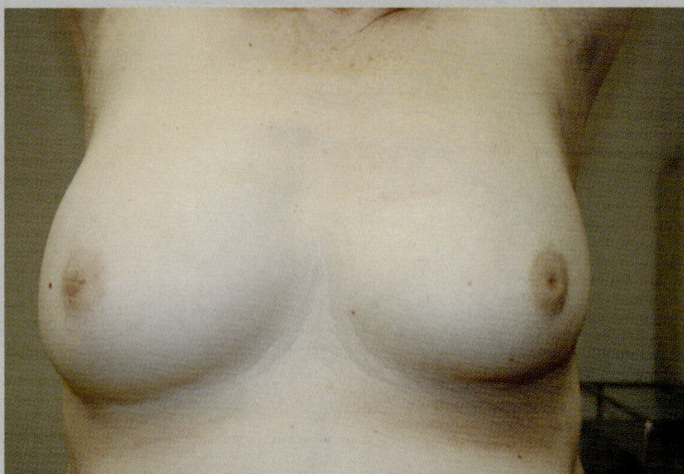

Image 3.1

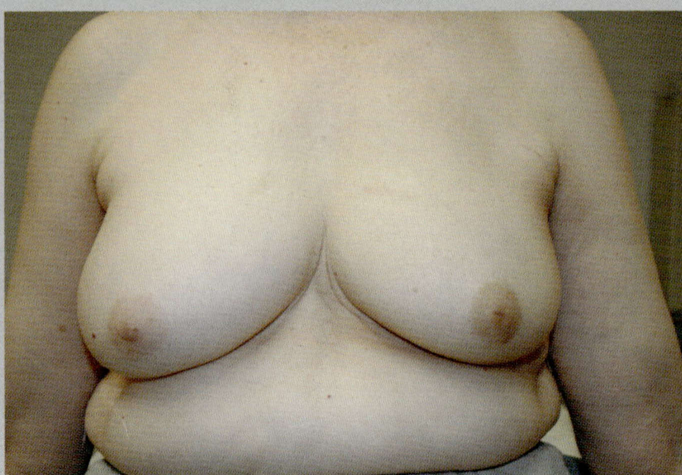

Image 3.2

### 7.1.2 *Radial Closure*

The breast tissue is approximated along a radial line. This kind of repair can be applied in any quadrant. It is particularly useful in the lower hemisphere of the breast between 3 o'clock and 9 o'clock [Figure 7.3(a–e)]. The resection is carried out as planned. We frequently shape the resection in an elliptical form to facilitate closure. After completion of the resection, the breast tissue is elevated off the pectoralis major fascia and rotated as in Figure 7.3(c). Both lateral and medial breast tissue are equally elevated and rotated when the tumor is located in the lower outer quadrant. For lesions in the inner lower quadrant, we have found that we frequently tend to mobilize the lateral flap to a greater extent than the medial flap, mainly due to the paucity of the breast tissue in the medial flap.

The breast tissue is approximated at multiple levels, starting with the deep layers and finishing with the surface of the breast [Figure 7.3(c–d)]. The skin is later approximated with subcuticular technique. In Figure 7.3(e), we have demonstrated a radial incision; this type of resection and repair could be completed through a transverse or even an inframammary incision. We certainly resort to a radial incision when we are planning to excise the skin overlying the tumor as presented in Case No. 4. Case No. 5 shows the final result of a patient after lumpectomy and axillary node dissection followed by chemotherapy and radiation for a T2 N1 palpable lesion located at the 9 o'clock axis of the left breast. The patient has A cup size breasts.

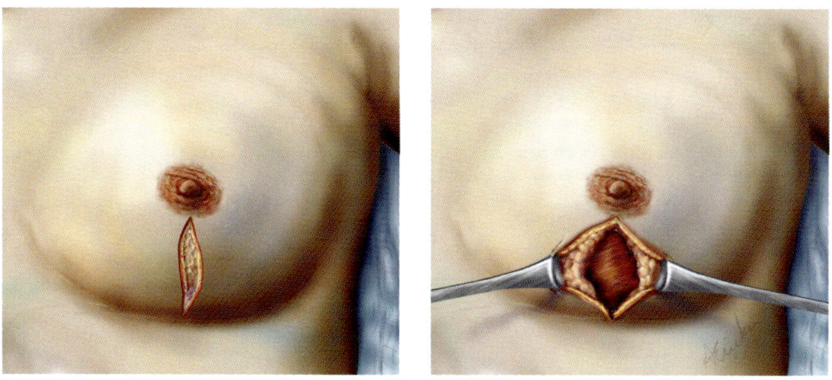

(a) (b)

Figure 7.3. (a–e) Radial closure of defects at 6 o'clock; (f–h) clinical example with 1-year postop.

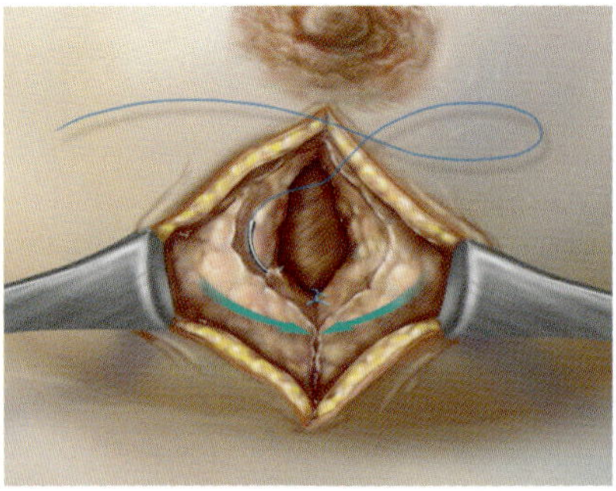

(c)

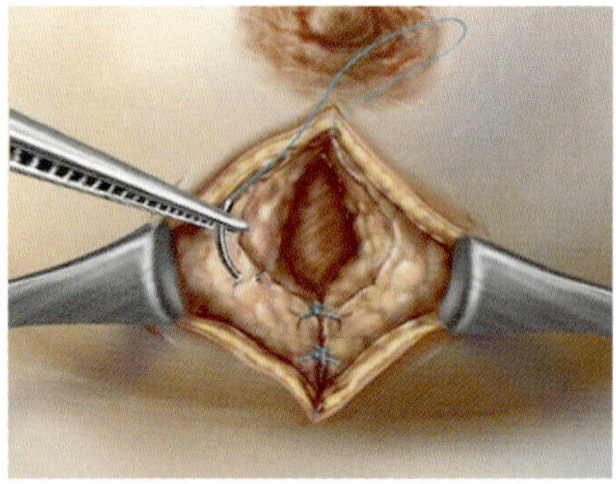

(d)

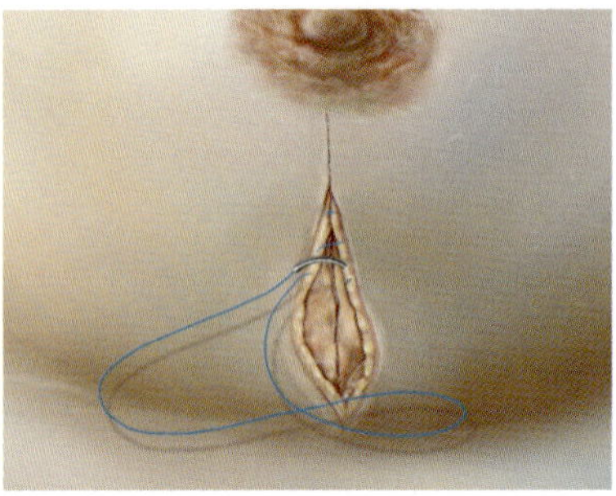

(e)

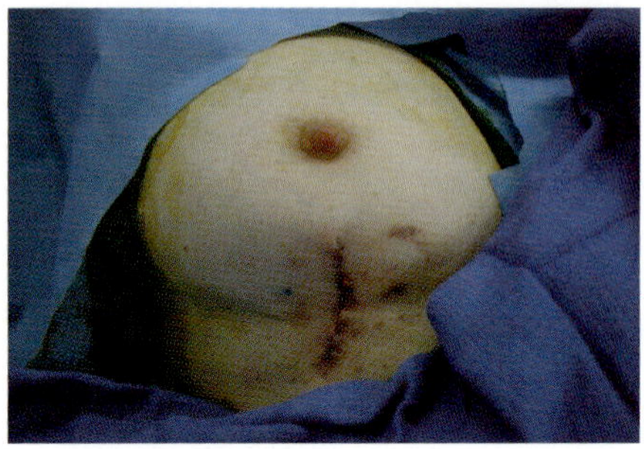

(f)

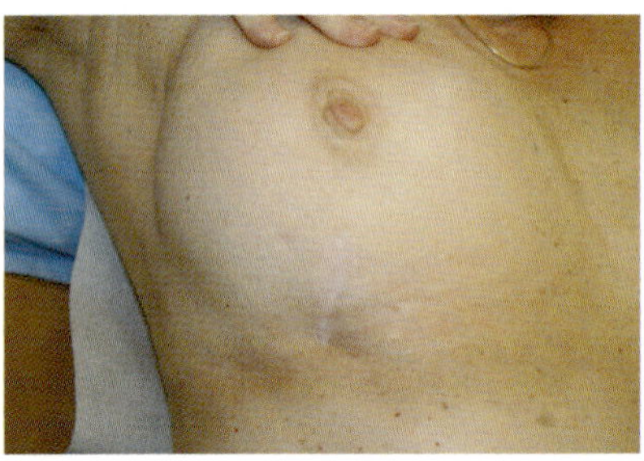

(g)

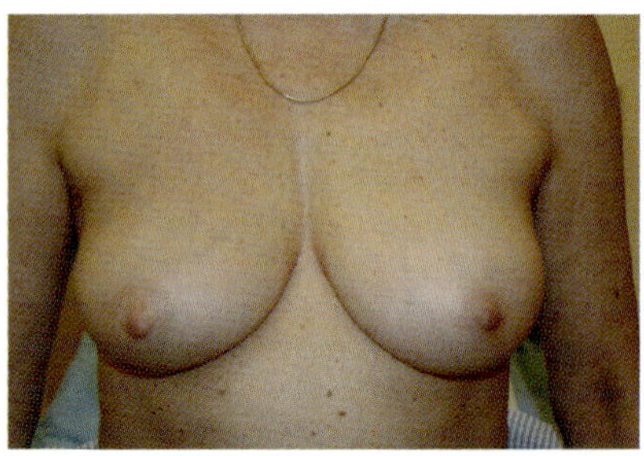

(h)

Figure 7.3. (*Continued*)

Case No. 4

Radial closure, inner lower quadrant. A 54-year-old woman presented with a palpable mass in the lower inner quadrant of the left breast. The tumor was close to the skin. We had planned a full-thickness resection of the skin, breast tissue down to the pectoralis fascia.

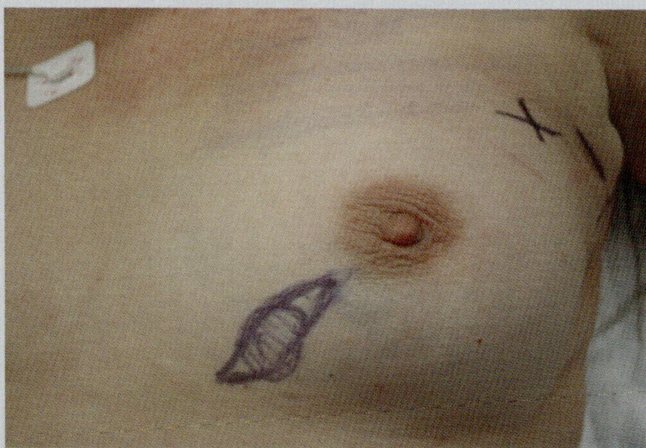

Image 4.1. The patient on the operating room table. The ellipse delineates the skin to be excised. The circle represents the underlying tumor.

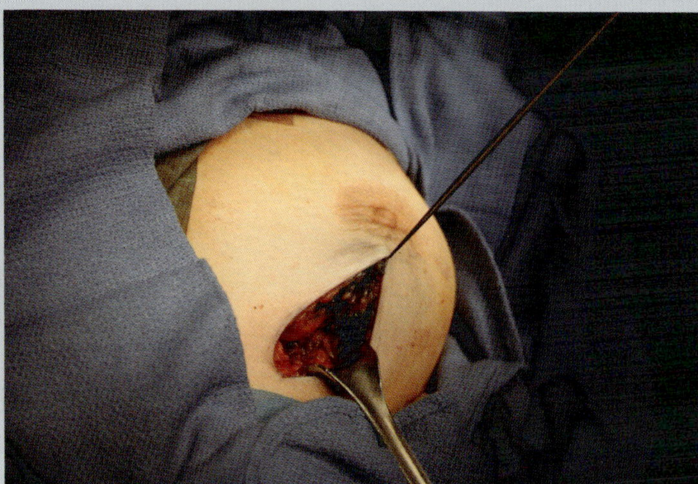

Image 4.2. The patient after resection of the skin and the tumor, and elevation of the glandular flaps, prior to rotation and approximation of the breast tissue.

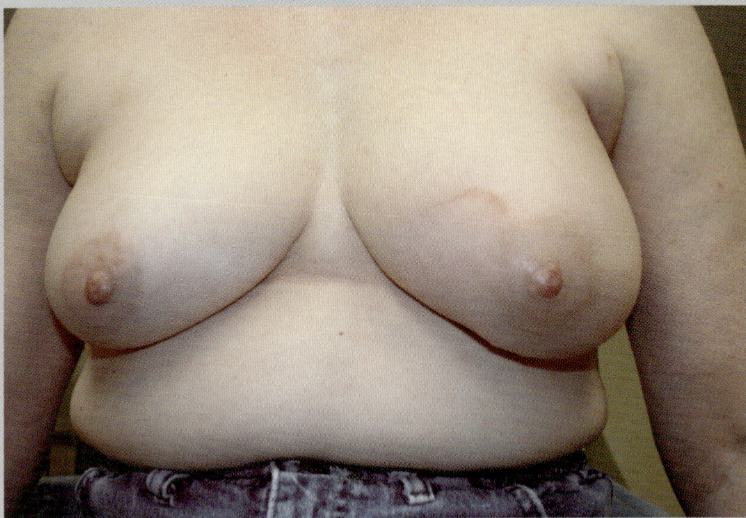

Image 4.3. The patient 10 days postoperatively. The reaction of the skin to the adhesive was still apparent. The operated breast is swollen and seems larger than the contralateral side.

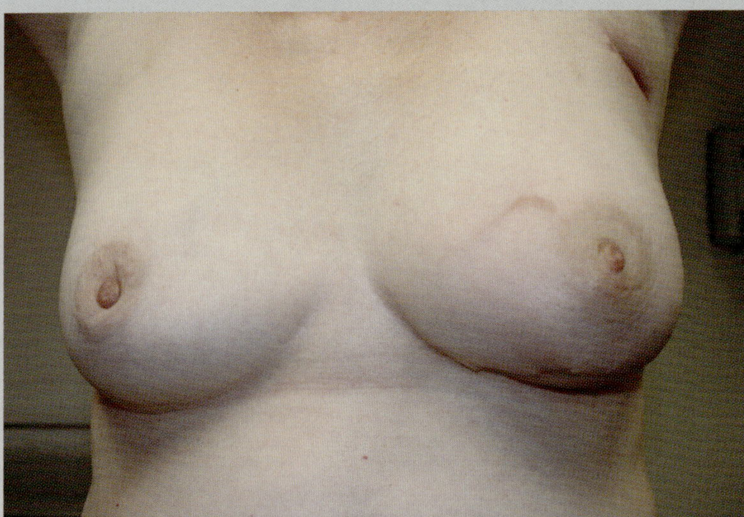

Image 4.4. Taken 10 days postoperatively with arm elevation. It is evident that the patient had loss of volume from the lower hemisphere, and the skin seems flattened due to the resection of an ellipse of skin.

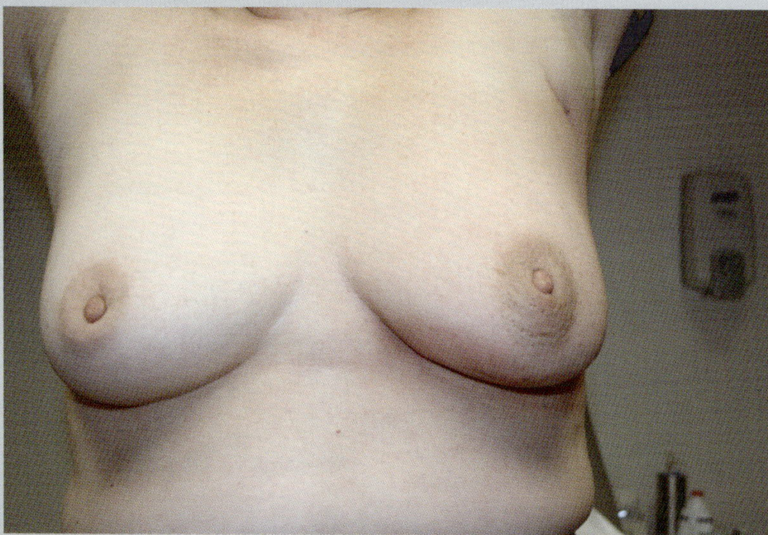

Image 4.5. Taken 8 months postoperatively after chemotherapy and completion of radiation treatment.

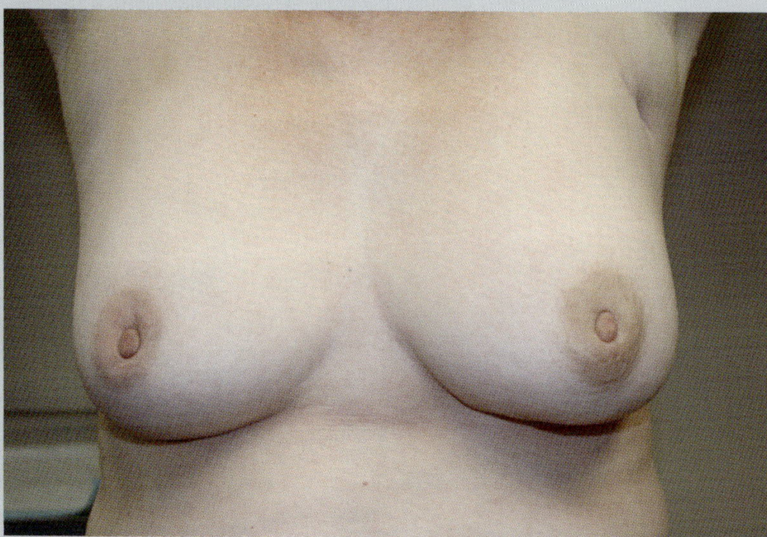

Image 4.6. Taken 1 year postoperatively. Note the excellent cosmetic results, symmetry in shape, and resolution of the flattening of the lower hemisphere.

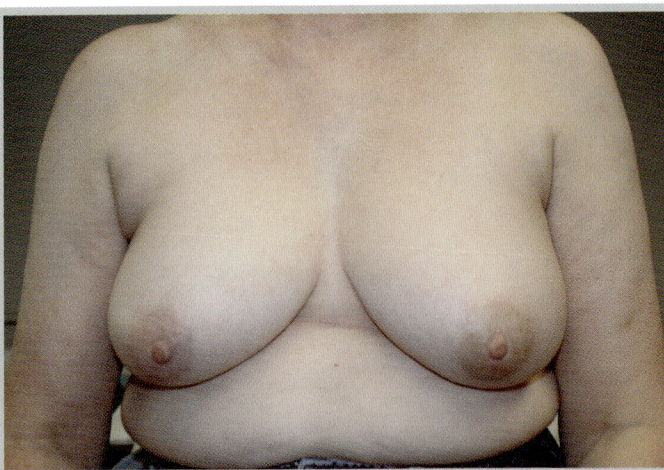

Image 4.7. Taken 1 year postoperatively as in Image 4.6.

Case No. 5

Radial closure, inner quadrant, left breast, 9 o'clock axis. A 48-year-old woman presented with a palpable mass in the 9 o'clock axis of the left breast. The tumor was around 2.4 cm in size and the patient had A cup size breasts. She underwent a lumpectomy and axillary node dissection. The defect was repaired along the 9 o'clock axis. The patient received a full course of chemotherapy and whole breast radiation with boost to the lumpectomy site.

- Images 5.1 and 5.2: The patient 6 years postoperatively. One clearly sees the difference in size, with the left breast smaller than the right. The shape of the left breast is within acceptable limits. The patient was extremely pleased with the cosmetic appearance of her operated side.

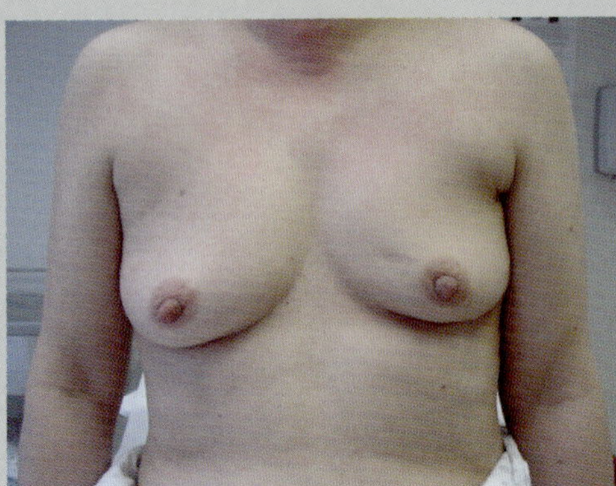

Image 5.1

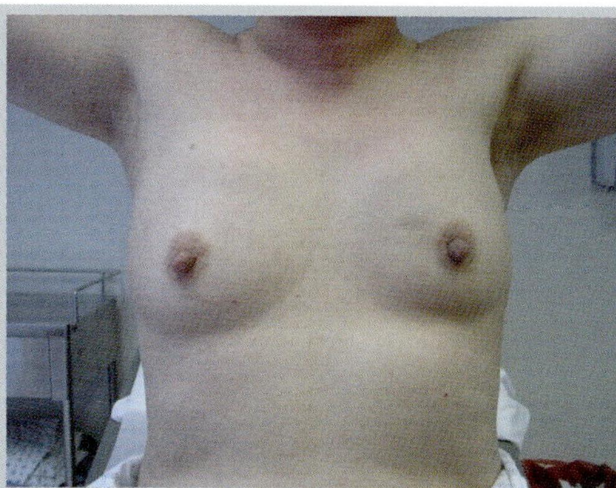

Image 5.2

### 7.1.3 *Triangular Closure (Also Known as "Mercedes" Closure)*

This is a combination of a transverse and radial repair. It is particularly useful in the upper hemisphere as it allows elevation of the NAC through the transverse segment but avoids displacement or malposition through the radial component. We have mostly used this type of repair in the upper outer quadrant to avoid outward deviation of the NAC.

As soon as the resection is completed, the defect is usually conical in shape. The repair is started by applying a triangular suture at the center of the defect [Figure 7.4(a)]. By tying that triangular suture, the walls of the defect are transformed into 3 lines [Figure 7.4(b)]. The breast tissue is approximated along these lines. The extent of elevation of the NAC is controlled by the initial triangular suture. Figure 7.5 shows how the surgeon can increase or decrease the extent of the elevation of the NAC by changing the position of the triangular suture. The extent of elevation is usually equal to a perpendicular line from point C to Line AB.

This kind of repair is also feasible through any skin incision. A key to the success of this repair is an adequate undermining of the overlying skin and mobilization of the breast tissue, particularly in patients with dense glandular tissue. Case No. 6 demonstrates the application of this technique in a patient with an upper outer quadrant lesion.

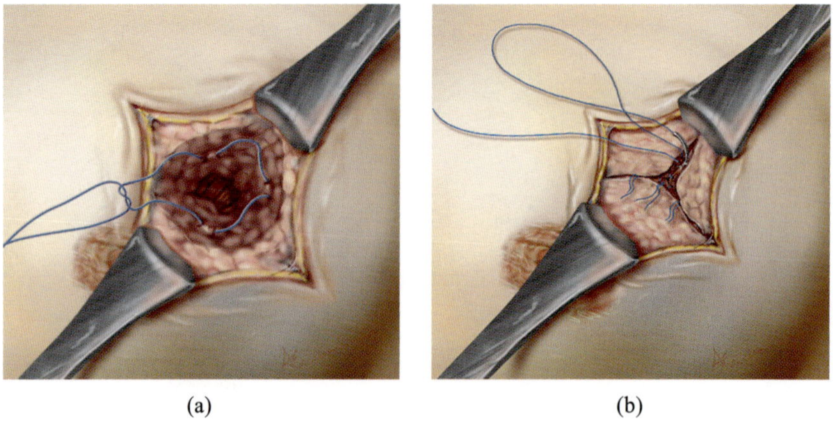


Figure 7.4. (a)–(b) Triangular repair.

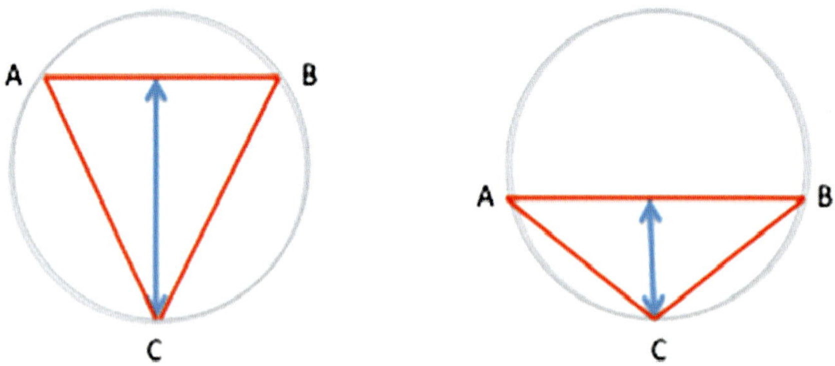


Figure 7.5. The surgeon can control the extent of NAC elevation by directly tuning the placement of the sutures at points A and B. The extent of elevation is equal to a perpendicular line from point C to the line AB.

Case No. 6

Triangular repair. A 41-year-old patient presented with a palpable mass in the upper outer quadrant of the right breast. She underwent a lumpectomy and axillary node dissection for a T2N1 breast cancer, followed by chemotherapy and radiation treatment. The resection involved a significant component of the UOQ. The repair was performed in a triangular fashion; the NAC was slightly elevated. However, it remained along the nipple line and matched very well with the contralateral side.

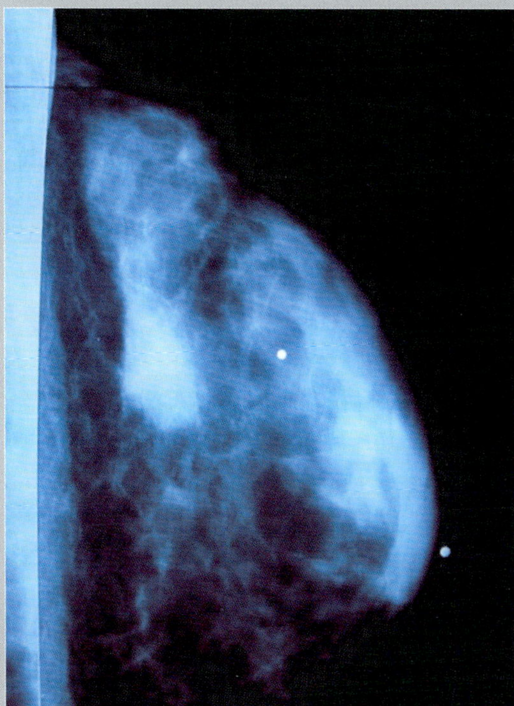

Image 6.1. The preoperative mammogram.

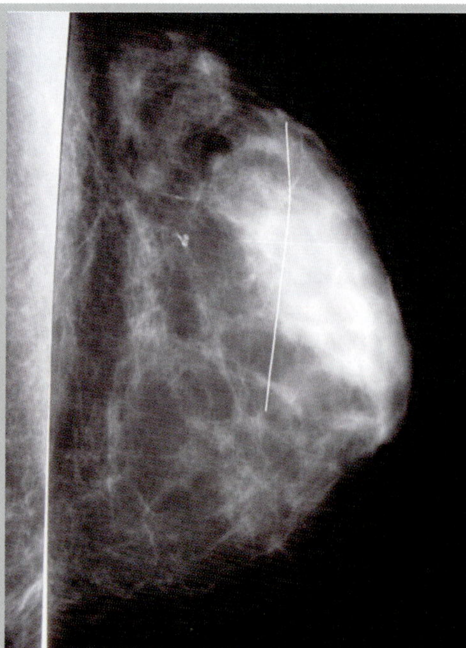

Image 6.2. The postoperative mammogram 3 years later. Note the calcification at the site of the tumor bed that represents the triangular suture. Note also the minimal scaring at the tumor site following the repair and closure of the defect. In patients in whom the tumor bed is left open, the scarring is significant and may result in some difficulty for early detection of any recurrences.

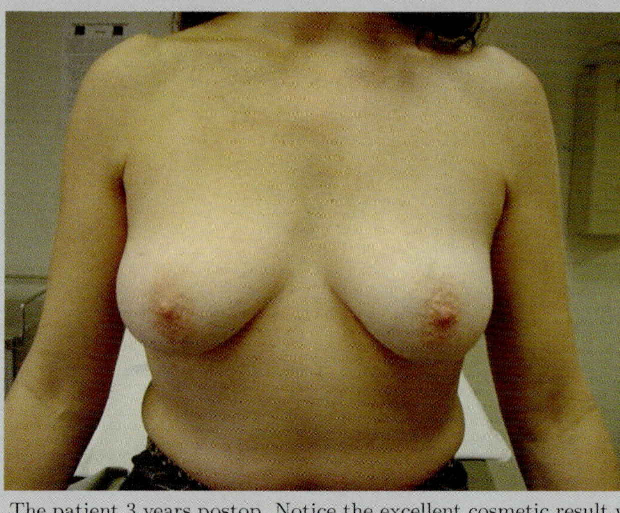

Image 6.3. The patient 3 years postop. Notice the excellent cosmetic result with subtle elevation of the NAC, and the perfect contour and projection of the operated breast.

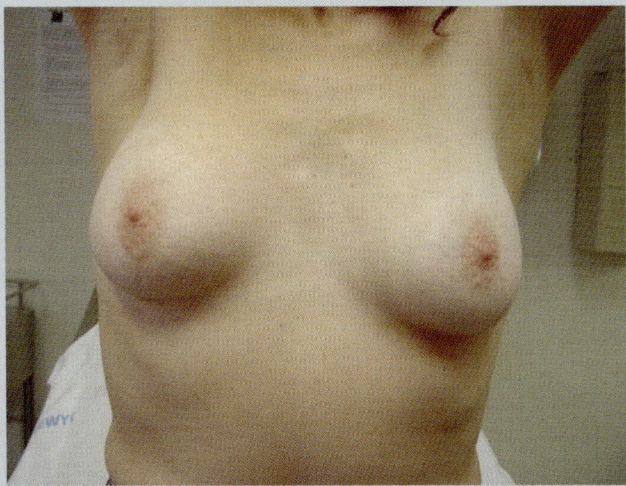

Image 6.4: The patient 3 years postop. Notice the excellent cosmetic result.

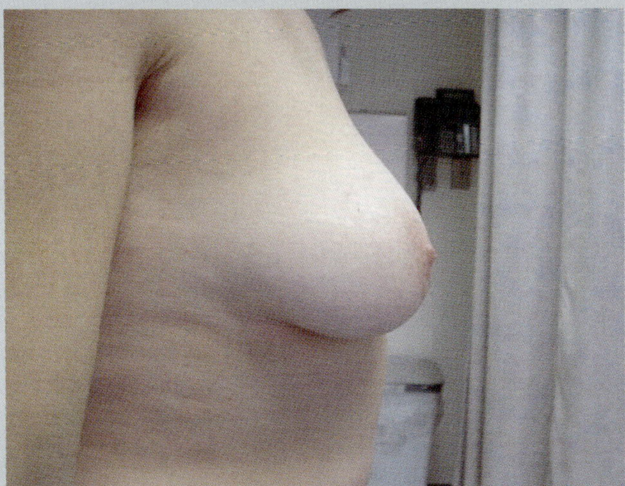

Image 6.5: The patient 3 years post-op. Notice the excellent cosmetic result and projection of the breast.

### 7.1.4 *Purse-String Closure*

We initially developed and applied this type of repair to terminal duct excision. So far, we have exclusively applied this repair to subareolar lesions. Theoretically, however, it could be applied to different parts of the breast as well. The NAC is elevated off the breast tissue, exposing the tissue to be resected. The thickness of the nipple areola flap directly depends on the

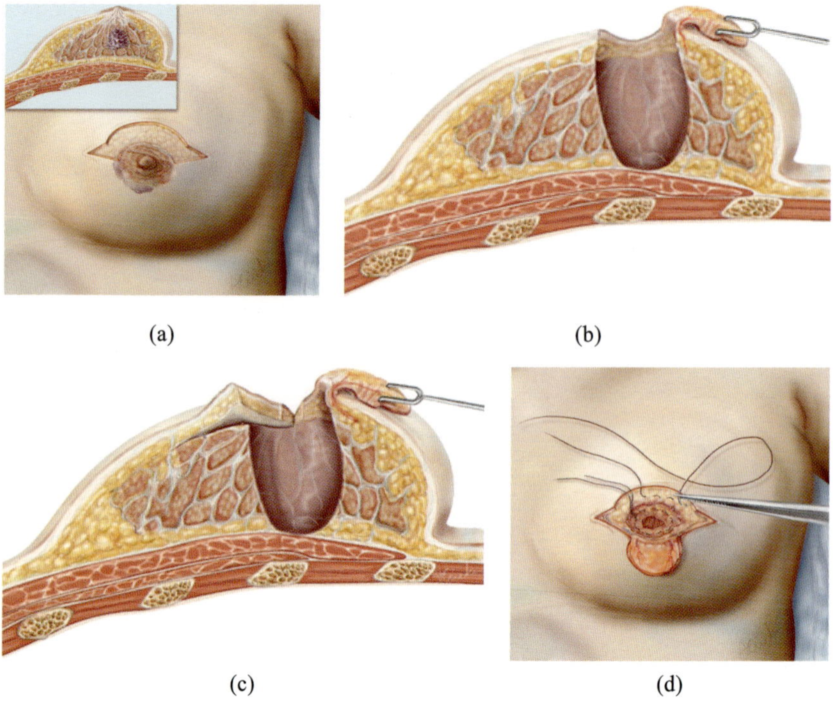

Figure 7.6. (a–d) Purse-string repair.

depth of the tumor. Again, when operating around the NAC, the surgeon has to be cognizant of the blood supply and innervation of that structure (see Chapter 1). The incision around the nipple areola should not extend beyond 50% of its circumference, and preferably less. If the diameter of the nipple areola is restrictive, we recommend extending the incision laterally or medially or to both sides for better exposure (Figure 7.6).

After elevation of the NAC, the resection is carried out as planned [Figure 7.6(b)]. This type of repair lends itself to resections that are circular or conical. It is our experience that in patients with large or fatty breasts, we may not need to extensively undermine the breast tissue off the pectoralis major muscle. It is, however, important to elevate the skin and subcutaneous tissue off the breast. This skin elevation should be limited to the cutaneous part of the incision; further undermining the skin where the NAC is attached may result in necrosis or denervation of that structure [Figure 7.6(c)]. We recommend resecting some of the skin above the NAC when a large resection of tissue under the NAC is required, as the NAC may appear wrinkled following approximation of the breast tissue. (Refer to Mastopexy Dome/Bat Wing Repair, Chapter 9.)

The repair is carried out by applying one or more purse-string sutures starting with the base of the defect [Figure 7.6(d)]. Case No. 7 shows the result of the technique applied in a patient with ductal carcinoma *in situ*.

Case No. 7

Purse-string repair. A 44-year-old woman with ductal carcinoma *in situ* in the center of the right breast. The patient underwent resection in the form of a terminal duct excision. We used the purse-string technique to repair the defect. The patient received postoperative radiation.

- Images 7.1–7.3 show the patient 4 years postoperatively.

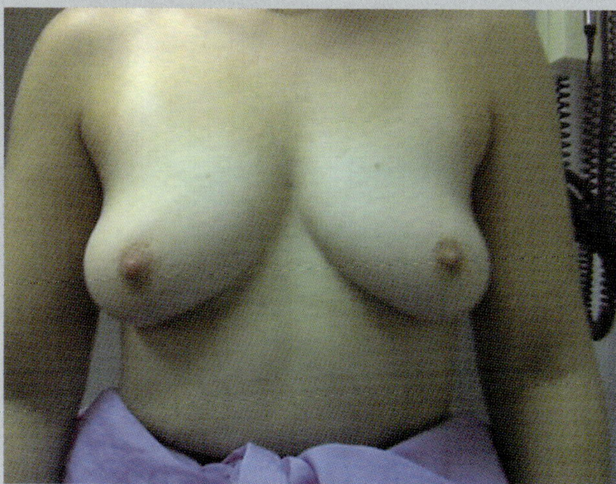

Image 7.1

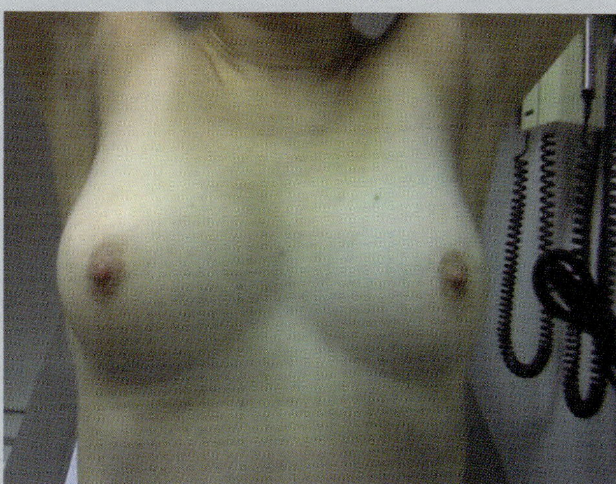

Image 7.2

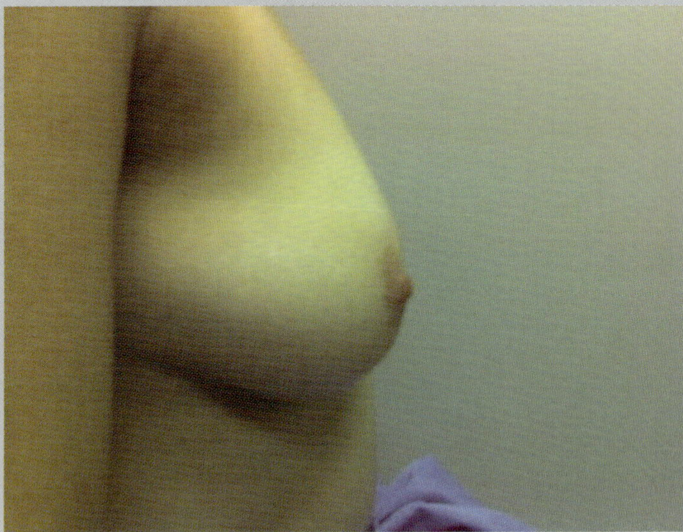

Image 7.3

### 7.1.5 *Mobilization of Surrounding Subcutaneous Tissue*

This type of repair is only possible when tumors are located around the periphery of the breast, particularly in the outer hemisphere. The prerequisite for this repair is the availability of contiguous tissue to be mobilized. The patient must have an excess of fat in the subcutaneous tissue surrounding the breast. The most common tissue we have used has been the lateral axillary fat pad and the subcutaneous tissue below the inframammary line. The resection is carried out routinely. The lateral axillary fat pad must be elevated off the serratus muscle and separated from the overlying skin. The axillary fat pad is then advanced and sutured to the breast tissue (Figure 7.7). The axillary fat pad may be directly advanced or rotated into the defect. We tend to minimally raise the breast tissue to avoid any lateral deviation of the NAC, and we mostly rely on the axillary fat pad to fill the defect. This technique could be combined with a partial transverse or radial repair of the glandular tissue. We strongly recommend elevating the fat pad off the serratus anterior muscle as the fat pad may retract in

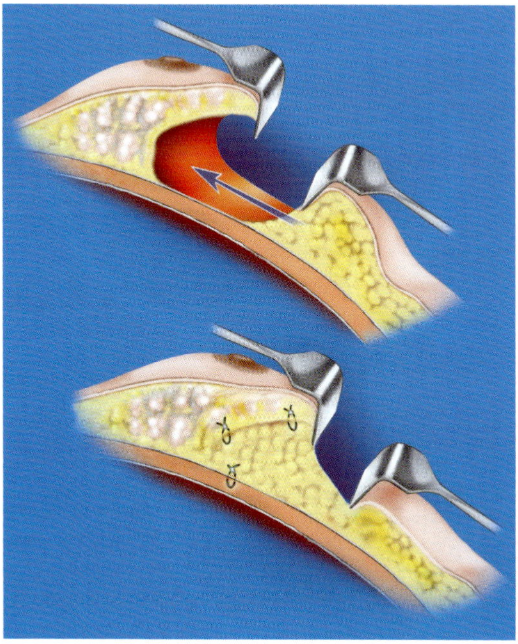

Figure 7.7. Mobilization of surrounding tissue.

the postoperative period. Case No. 8 demonstrates the application of this technique.

Case No. 8
This is a 68-year-old woman who had right breast cancer treated with breast conservation. While on aromatase inhibitors, she presented with a left invasive lobular carcinoma estrogen receptor positive and progesterone receptor positive tumor, involving a significant segment of the outer quadrant between 2 o'clock and 4 o'clock. The patient insisted on breast conservation. She had multiple medical problems and was not a candidate for neoadjuvant chemotherapy.

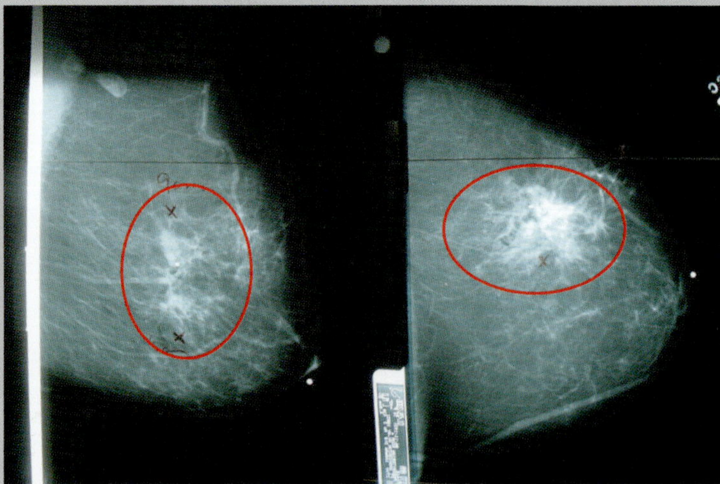

Image 8.1. The preoperative mammogram and the extent of resection, estimated preoperatively.

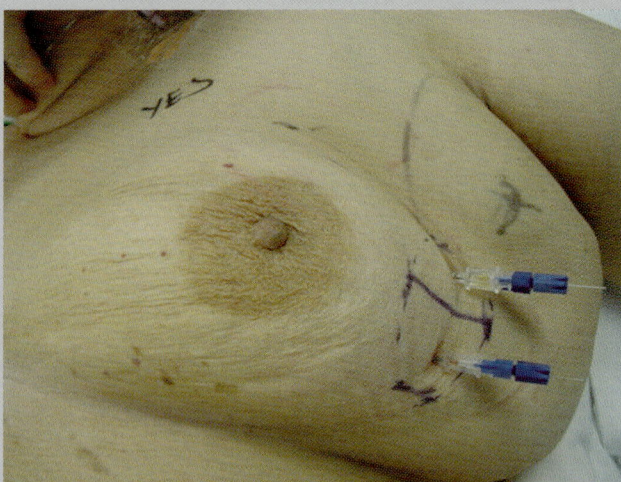


Image 8.2. The patient on the operating table with needle localization wires bracketing the lesion. Note the extent of the axillary fat pad that could be used to repair the defect.

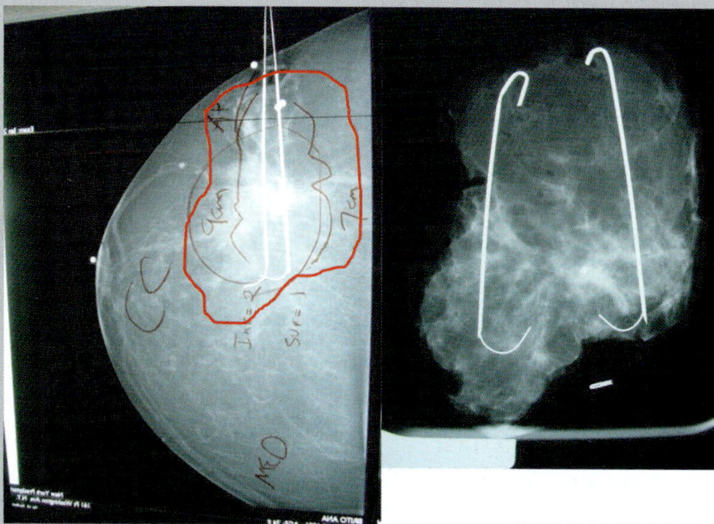

Image 8.3. The patient mammogram after the needle localization, and the specimen radiogram showing the extent of resection.

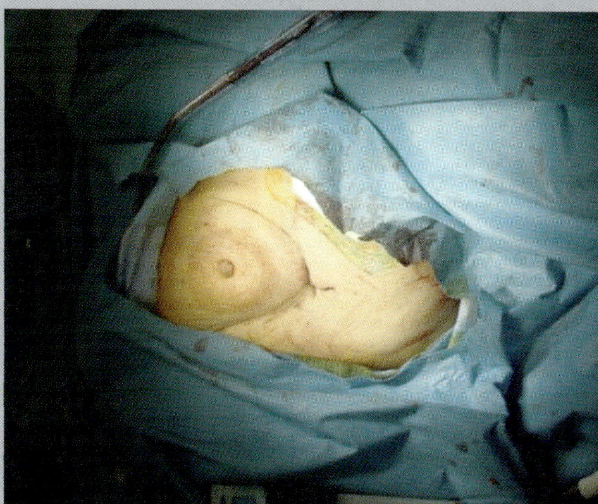

Image 8.4. On the operating table, we approximated the subcutaneous tissue without repairing the defect. Note the resulting extensive depression and adherence of the skin to the chest wall.

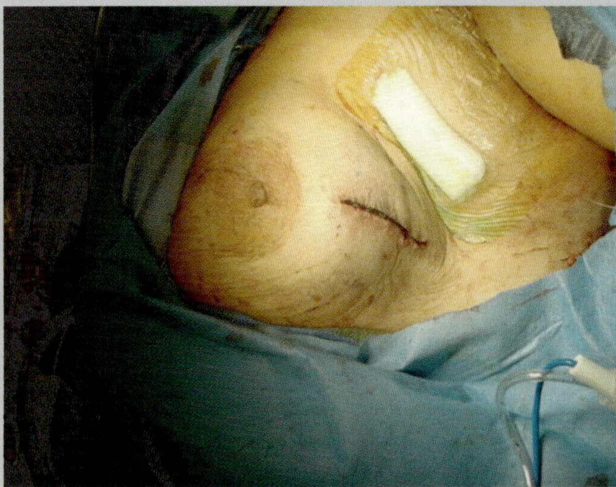

Image 8.5. The patient after completion of the repair and approximation of the subcutaneous tissue. It is obvious that the repair has filled the defect preventing the depression of the skin and restored the contours of the breast. Also note the loss of the lateral fat pad that has been mobilized to repair the defect.

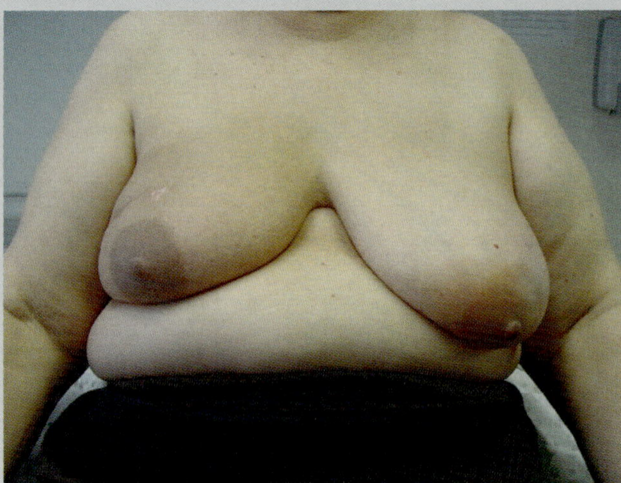

Image 8.6. The patient in the postoperative period. The right breast shows the effect of prior radiation. The left breast contours are maintained.

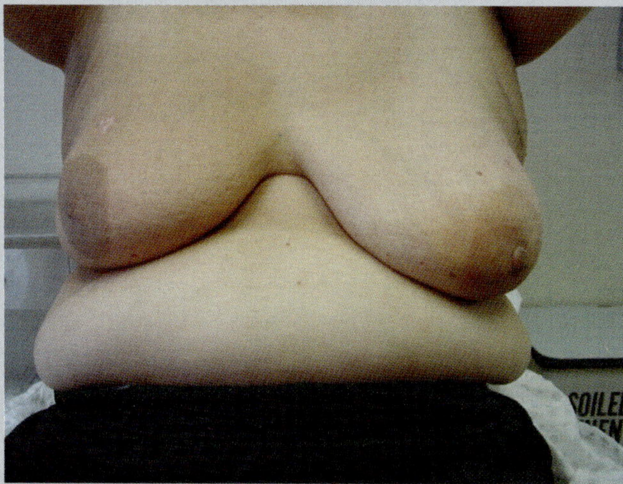

Image 8.7. The patient in the postoperative period as in Image 8.6.

These techniques are simple easy to learn and apply. Regardless of the technique you use, we recommend the following important steps:

- Orient the specimen to facilitate limited re-excision as needed, thus avoiding re-excision of the totality of the cavity.
- Apply clips to the wall of the defect prior to initiating the repair.
- Document the steps used to repair the defect in the operative note. The operative note will be a useful document when patient returns to the operating room for re-excision of margins.

## References

1. Bostwick J. (1983) *Correction of Breast Asymmetries. Aesthetic and Reconstructive Breast Surgery.* Mosby Company, St. Louis, Toronto, London, p. 252.

## Chapter 8

# ONCOPLASTIC BREAST REDUCTION

Tara L. Huston,* Christine H. Rohde,* Mahmoud El-Tamer,† and Jeffrey Ascherman*

**Division of Plastic Surgery, New York-Presbyterian Hospital/Columbia University Medical Center, New York, NY, USA*

*†Breast Service, Department of Surgery, Memorial Sloan-Kettering Cancer Center, New York, NY, USA*

## 8.1 Introduction

Improved survival, coupled with enhanced patient expectations, created the impetus for better aesthetic results in breast-conservation therapy (BCT). This driving force has encouraged breast surgeons and plastic surgeons to work together to design operations that are oncologically sound and maximize the cosmetic outcome.[1]

Over the past 2 decades, there has been an increase in the number of women with breast cancer who are treated with BCT. BCT is a combination of local tumor resection and breast radiation therapy, which allows a woman to keep her breast. It has an equivalent disease-free survival when compared to traditional mastectomy. This increase in BCT is a result of increased screening and earlier mammography, and a corresponding increase in small, early-stage breast cancers. Also, it is important to note the increased use of neoadjuvant chemotherapy (NCT), which drastically decreases tumor size, thus permitting breast-conserving procedures. Lastly, the desire of many women to preserve their breast for psychological reasons, regardless of cosmetic outcome, has led to greater use of BCT.

It is well established that local control of breast cancer may affect survival and that clear margins are warranted when breast preservation is undertaken. From the National Surgical Adjuvant Breast and

Bowel Project (NSABP) B-06 trial, it is known that long-term survival is comparable for patients who undergo total mastectomy as well as those who choose BCT.[2] It is also known that there is a small decrease in deaths from breast cancer in patients who undergo lumpectomy and radiation instead of just lumpectomy. The goals of BCT are both ablative and reconstructive in nature. They include an oncologically sound resection of tumor, radiation of the resection bed, and preservation of the breast for an aesthetic outcome that is, in theory, superior to a mastectomy.

Resection of large volumes of breast tissue, however, may result in poor aesthetic outcomes. Patients may be left with significant breast asymmetry, scarring, and deformity. This would negate a central purpose of BCT. Up to 30% of patients who have undergone BCT end up with poor cosmetic results.[3,4] Suboptimal surgical results are then further compromised by necessary irradiation. The number may be even higher as some women are too self-conscious or frustrated to seek further consultation or surgery to improve their breast appearance. Correction of these deformities can involve multiple challenges made only more difficult by the use of irradiated tissues. However, it is important not to compromise the tenets of sound oncologic management to obtain an optimal cosmetic outcome.

## 8.2 The Oncoplastic Approach

Aesthetic techniques were merged with oncologic treatments in the 1990s.[5] The first study of lower-pole tumors in which the breast reduction included the tumor was published in 1990.[6] The term "oncoplastic breast surgery" was coined in the mid-1990s.[7] The oncoplastic concept is based on the ability to perform large oncologic resections while adhering to the principles of aesthetic breast reduction surgery. It was developed to anticipate, and take steps to prevent, these poor outcomes at the time of the ablative surgery. With the addition of oncoplastic techniques, the rate of poor aesthetic outcomes can be reduced to below 7%.[8] In addition to aesthetic advantages, there are oncologic advantages to the oncoplastic approach. Some studies have demonstrated higher frequency of negative margins and less-frequent return to the operating room when comparing standard lumpectomy to oncoplastic lumpectomy in large tumors.[9]

Cochrane *et al.* demonstrated that as much as 10% of the glandular volume of a breast can be removed without significant cosmetic deformity. Also, the larger a breast is, the more tolerant it is to resection.[10] Clough stated that up to 25% of the breast may be excised; however, local parenchymal rearrangement or skin excision is necessary for satisfactory results.[11] With this logic, it would make sense that oncoplastic breast surgery is indicated for patients who are able to reduce the volume of their breasts in excess of 20% to 25%. It is also a useful tool for difficult tumor locations, such as the inner quadrants, centrally, and along the inframammary fold (IMF) where small resections without local tissue rearrangement may be deforming.

It is estimated that up to 40% of women treated with BCT begin with a breast size that could be categorized as macromastia.[12] Even though there is a seemingly ideal breast-to-tumor ratio in these women, this population tends to suffer more complications. The cosmesis is often unsatisfactory as irradiating a large, ptotic breast can lead to a heterogeneous dose distribution. This is a result of repeated positioning over a prolonged course of treatment.[13] Breast size does affect cosmetic outcome, with larger-breasted women faring worse. In addition, attempting surgical correction of irradiated tissue to correct the cosmetic issue is fraught with complications. For these women with macromastia, the combined oncoplastic approach has the benefit of relieving symptoms, as well as treating the cancer.[14]

In summary, using the oncoplastic approach of reduction mammaplasty can make it easier to obtain the desired oncologic and cosmetic outcomes. It affords the surgeons a large incision, with possible access to the axilla, thus possibly preventing a second incision. It prophylaxes against cosmetic sequelae, such as breast asymmetry, and may even relieve symptoms of macromastia in certain patients. Smaller breast size may also translate to improved radiation therapy (RT) efficiency. Also, the reduction allows tissue sampling of the contralateral breast and provides a theoretical risk reduction through removal of excess breast parenchyma. Occult breast cancers have been reported in up to 4% of contralateral symmetrizing reduction specimens in patients undergoing breast reconstruction.[15]

It is important that the ablative surgeon understands the concepts of breast aesthetics, volume, and symmetry, and be cognizant of when preoperative referral to a plastic surgeon might be beneficial. In turn, it is critical that the reconstructive surgeon understands the tenets of oncologic surgery and is able to devise an operative plan that does not violate them. Communication between the ablative and reconstructive surgeon is vital.

## 8.3 Patient Selection and Preoperative Breast Evaluation

Patient selection depends on a number of factors, the most important of which are a patient's desire for a smaller breast and the cancer surgeon's concern about creating a cosmetic deformity while obtaining adequate specimen size. The ideal candidate is a patient who has symptoms of macromastia, such as chronic headaches, back pain, neck pain, shoulder grooving, or intertriginous rashes, and who requires a large-volume resection, although any patient with moderate-to-large–sized breasts can be considered. The goal is to provide a survival rate comparable to standard BCT, a good aesthetic outcome, and enhanced patient satisfaction.[16] In plastic surgery practices, women who have had breast reduction tend to express higher patient satisfaction as the reduction in breast volume and weight allows them to wear new clothing and embark upon new activities hitherto impossible.

The use of reduction mammaplasty has been ongoing for almost 200 years. It is only recently that we have combined the procedure with ablative breast surgery. Surgeons have performed reduction mammaplasty since the 1840s, which then consisted of removal of excess breast parenchyma and skin via the IMF.[17] The classic goals of breast reduction are to improve symptomatology, decrease the volume of breast tissue without impairing vascular and nerve supply to the nipple areola complex (NAC), reposition the NAC to an anatomically correct position, create a better breast shape, provide parenchymal support for a long-lasting result, and discard excess skin and minimize scarring.[18]

After the patient makes the decision to undergo breast reconstruction after lumpectomy, the surgical team must contemplate the time course. Immediate reconstruction is psychologically and aesthetically preferable. In some patients, however, delay may be prudent. Younger patients with extensive ductal carcinoma *in situ* (DCIS) are not good candidates for a 1-stage approach as there is a high rate of positive margins. Reconstruction in these women should be deferred until confirmation of negative margins. This is one group of patients who should be counseled preoperatively about a 2-stage procedure.[16]

There are 2 breasts involved in the decision-making process, and the treatment plan must take this into account. It is agreed upon that in the vast majority of cases, immediate breast reconstruction can be undertaken on the breast that has just undergone a resection. The cases in which a delay is preferable were just mentioned. Symmetry is crucial in obtaining a good cosmetic outcome. Many surgeons will reduce or symmetrize the contralateral breast at the first procedure in order to spare the patient a second operation. However, it is impossible to know the final size of the ipsilateral breast following cancer ablation; therefore, the size and shape of the contralateral breast is an educated approximation. Fitoussi *et al.* actually demonstrated a shift from synchronous reconstruction in the early years to delayed contralateral symmetrizing reduction in the later years of their 540-case study.[19]

Patient counseling is an integral part of the preoperative work-up. With a traditional lumpectomy, positive margins on final pathology often warrant a re-excision of the resection cavity. After an oncoplastic reduction, the "cavity" out of which the specimen was removed no longer exists as it did at resection. During the reduction mammaplasty procedure, its geometry is altered significantly so that margins cannot be identified. As such, if the margins are positive following an oncoplastic reduction, a total mastectomy may be the necessary next step. Encouragingly, however, a larger volume of breast tissue can be removed with the oncoplastic procedure, thus making the theoretical risk of positive margins smaller. Additionally, patients must understand that nipple complications from the ablation, reduction, and subsequent radiation are possible. This may mean decreased sensation, and partial or total thickness skin loss, as well as wound-healing issues (see Case No. 2, Image 2.4).

## 8.4 History and Physical

A detailed history and physical are necessary. In the history, it is important to elicit issues pertaining to macromastia, such as chronic headaches, back pain, neck pain, shoulder grooving, or intertriginous rashes, as well as a personal and family history of breast surgery, cancers, connective tissue diseases, and radiation to the thorax. A history of smoking predisposes to increased flap necrosis, and efforts must be taken to help the patient quit immediately if she is currently smoking.

On examination, height and weight should be measured, and a body mass index can then be calculated. There should be emphasis on breast size, shape, prior scars, degree of ptosis, and position of the lesion. The most commonly used system to classify breast ptosis includes 3 grades: grade 1 is mild, with the nipple at the IMF; grade 2 is moderate, with the nipple below the IMF, but with lower-pole tissue below the nipple; grade 3 is severe, with the nipple well below the IMF and no lower-pole tissue below it. Pseudoptosis is actually inferior pole ptosis with the nipple at or above the IMF, which is often seen in postpartum breast atrophy. Measurements may be taken of the breast width, sternal notch-to-nipple distance, nipple-to-inframammary–fold distance, and NAC width (see Chapter 2). Asymmetries should be documented and pointed out to the patient. Preoperative photographs may also be taken at this time.

## 8.5 Types of Breast Reduction

A team approach is crucial for the success of excising a breast lesion in combination with a breast reduction. The breast and plastic surgeon should clearly communicate preoperatively to define the areas to be excised, thus allowing the plastic surgeons to design their reduction techniques. A good result requires a thorough knowledge of basic mammaplasty techniques. The choice of incision and pedicle depend on a number of factors. The most important determinant is the tumor location; however, one must also consider the location of previous scars/needle biopsy sites, and whether these need to be excised, as well as the need for access to the axilla. Excision of the skin overlying the tumor and its extent, although not always needed, has to be taken into consideration and clearly defined preoperatively. Surgeon comfort with the various types of reduction mammaplasties is a factor as well. When designing the operation, consideration must also be given to the potential for radiation and how this may alter the eventual size of the breast. Radiation can lead to chronic edema, as well as involution or shrinkage of the remaining breast tissue. The combined approach of excising a tumor and reducing the breast is applicable to patients who present without any prior surgical intervention or after an attempt at breast conservation with positive margins.

## 8.6 Relevant Anatomy

The blood supply to the breast comes primarily from the internal thoracic artery through its anterior perforators, as well as the lateral thoracic artery, thoracoacromial artery, and the lateral perforators of the intercostal arteries. The NAC receives contributions from all of those vessels (see Chapter 1).

Nerve supply to the NAC arises from the anterior and lateral perforating branches of the third, fourth, and fifth intercostal nerves. The fourth intercostal branch is thought to be the primary sensory contributor. In order to maintain sensibility of the NAC, it is important to avoid violation of the pectoralis fascia along the deep lateral resection margin. Interestingly, some women have increased sensitivity postoperatively, possibly from reduced traction on the nerve with a lighter postoperative breast. Medially, the nerve branches lie more superficially. Therefore, maintenance of the dermoparenchymal relationship anteromedially, which is done with the superomedial pedicle, may help to decrease the potential for injury to these superficial nerves during pedicle dissection and rotation (see Chapter 1).

Breast dimensions and degrees of ptosis, recorded in the history and physical, can also assist in making the decision regarding which type of surgery to perform. In the 1950s Penn defined breast aesthetics by studying 150 healthy women, 20 of whom had "perfect" breasts. He found that an equilateral triangle existed between the suprasternal notch and both nipples whose limbs are approximately 21 cm in length. He also found this to be the distance from the mid-clavicular line to the nipple. In this study, the average nipple-to-IMF distance was 6.9 cm.[20] Although these are not absolutes, as patients and their breasts come in all shapes and sizes, the symmetry is a useful guide to keep in mind (see Chapter 2).

## 8.7 Technical Considerations

The first and key goal of this oncoplastic approach is to achieve the most complete and appropriate resection of the cancer with histologically negative margins. It has been well documented that a positive margin is associated with significantly higher incidence of local recurrence.[21,22]

Knowledge of margin status is important prior to embarking on an immediate reconstruction. Intraoperative assessments of the margins are advisable when the breast surgeon is not confident about the extent of resection. We recommend gross examination of the specimen, and the surgeon can also consider radiologic imaging. Specimen mammogram with two 90-degree images is quite helpful for assessment of microcalcifications. Currently, some surgeons have noticed a drop in their re-excision rate with intraoperative ultrasound, particularly with solid masses.[23,24]

Histologic evaluation is also helpful in cases involving large tumors. Frozen sections with touch preparation are one of the most accepted current methods of intraoperative histologic assessment of margins. Newer technologies are currently being evaluated, such as Spectroscopy or the MarginProbe (Dune Medical Devices, Caesarea, Israel), which is a recently developed device for real-time intraoperative margin assessment.[25] Pleijhuis *et al.* have described the current modalities and future directions in assessing surgical margins.[26] It is well known that local recurrence is proportional to the size of the tumor, as well as the positive or negative margin status at the initial resection.[27] Clear margins may be difficult to confirm at the initial operation for women with infiltrating lobular cancer or in multicentric or multifocal DCIS. The breast surgeon has to achieve a histologically negative margin. The definition of a histologically negative margin has been extensively debated in the literature. Chapter 5 in this book has an extensive review of the literature and presents an evidence-based recommendation. Each surgeon or institution has specific guidelines as to what constitutes an appropriate margin, and we recommend they be followed.

It has often been our practice, particularly following a major oncoplastic approach, to mark the margins of resection with hemoclips. The clips will be used by the radiation oncologist as a guide for RT, particularly for the appropriate delivery of a boost dose.

Once the preoperative evaluation is complete and the timing has been selected, there are 2 major decisions to make when designing a breast reduction. The first is the location and size of the incision, and the second is the origin of the dermoglandular pedicle on which the nipple will rest.

## 8.8 Incision

There are a myriad of options for the incision; however, the 2 most commonly used are the Wise pattern or inverted "T", and the vertical. The inverted "T" pattern incision travels along the IMF and traverses centrally up to the nipple — hence the name. It allows wide access to the breast parenchyma and can be used with any pedicle, for a tumor in any location; also, it permits skin excision in both the vertical and horizontal dimensions for optimal breast shaping. Depending on the pedicle and the desire to avoid wide undermining, a separate small incision may be needed in the axilla for lymph node sampling or clearance. The Wise pattern, or inverted "T", is the most commonly used incision for oncoplastic breast reductions. For a woman to be a candidate for an oncoplastic breast reduction, she will most likely have both excess tissue and excess skin. The Wise pattern is ideal for women who need skin and tissue excision in both the vertical and the horizontal dimensions, leaving the surgeon the most opportunities for breast reshaping (see Chapter 2).

The vertical scar mammaplasty was introduced by Lassus[28] and modified by Lejour.[29] This incision travels around the NAC and extends down to the IMF (see Chapter 2). Although the access to the breast parenchyma is good, the axilla is not easily reached. The vertical scar technique only allows for breast skin reduction in the horizontal axis. The vertical size reduction is achieved through a cinching closure of the skin. In the classic Lejour breast reduction, the volume is also decreased with liposuction, but it would be advisable to avoid this step in a cancer operation. This incision is employed when the surgeon or the patient wishes to minimize the scar as much as possible, while resecting a large volume of breast parenchyma. Some surgeons believe that the long-term downside of this approach is the tendency of the inferior pole of the newly reconstructed breast to bottom out over time as the skin envelope stretches.

The periareolar approach, based on Benelli's "round block" technique, leaves an incision that is solely around the nipple and does not extend out onto the breast (See Chapter 9, Figure 9.9).[30] This provides good access to the upper pole; however, it does not permit a great deal of skin excision. It is useful for women with mild ptosis in whom a mastopexy might be considered, but is not a good option when volume reduction is required. In the majority of women who are candidates for an oncoplastic reduction mammaplasty, a large volume reduction is required; as a result, this is not a commonly utilized option.

The lateral mammaplasty is similar to the vertical; however, the scar runs from the nipple laterally out toward the anterior axillary line (see Chapter 9, Figures 9.7–9.11). This incision is suitable for lateral tumors. Bearing in mind that the majority of breast tumors are located laterally, this is an important approach. A benefit to this technique is the avoidance of thin, large surface-area dermal flaps. It creates thick flaps that are more tolerant to radiation. This incision may be extended superiorly to gain access to the axilla. The medial mammaplasty is the reverse of the lateral mammaplasty, with the incision heading toward the sternum, and is most useful for medial tumors (see Chapter 9: Case 2 and Figure 9.12).[31]

The omegaplasty, also referred to as the bat-wing excision, is a transverse scar above and alongside the nipple which is not aesthetically ideal; however, it provides good access to superomedially located tumors.[32] This is a challenging area because there is little breast volume to begin with in repose, and even less after ablative resection. No undermining is required with this incision, which is a plus for radiation, but it does little to decrease breast volume or address ptosis. If too much skin and parenchyma are resected with this incision superior to the nipple, it may result in pseudoptosis (see Chapter 9: Case 1 and Figure 9.4).

The IMF plasty, similar to the very first breast reductions performed in the 19th Century, places an incision along the IMF. There is no vertical extension. This is good for a narrow breast that only requires reduction in the vertical dimension. Oftentimes, the periareolar scar and nipple dissection can be avoided with this technique. This method will decrease the nipple-to-inframammary–fold distance. If it is already short, then superior transposition of the nipple and creation of a periareolar scar may be necessary.

## 8.9 Pedicle

The other decision that needs to be made is pedicle position. The pedicle is the dermoglandular tissue on which the vascular and nervous supply to the nipple is carried. The most commonly used pedicles are inferior, superior, and medial. The superolateral pedicle is less commonly used, but is an excellent choice for lower, inner tumors.[33] The other option, rarely used in cosmetic surgery but needed for reconstruction after extirpation of medial tumors, is the lateral pedicle. All have their cosmetic and sensory advantages and disadvantages. The decision of which one to use for non-oncologic breast surgery is often based on surgeon preference. However, in oncoplastic breast-reduction surgery, the pedicle is, by necessity, chosen based on what remains following the ablation of the tumor. For example, a lower-pole tumor will clear out the glandular tissue in the lower half of the breast so the reconstructive surgeon will be left to choose between the various superior pedicles.

The superior pedicle is solid, reliable, and may better preserve nipple sensation. Innervation to the nipple is superficial and descends from the clavicular area, thus preserving sensation. This pedicle, however, is limited by difficulty in moving the nipple long distances, especially in patients with significant breast hypertrophy. This is a challenging pedicle to undertake with a large reduction, as molding the breast into an aesthetically pleasing shape may be difficult with only superior fullness. However, this is a good pedicle to use for lower quadrant tumors, especially in moderate-sized breasts.

The medial or superomedial pedicle is increasingly popular in aesthetic breast surgery. It is shorter than the other pedicles and requires rotation, not folding, for its inset. Sensory innervation comes from the anterior rami of the intercostal nerves. Due to its orientation and rotation, the medial pedicle is excellent for retaining breast shape. This pedicle can be used for a tumor in the lower quadrants, or laterally on the breast. This is an increasingly popular choice in non-oncologic breast reductions in that regard, as well as in regards to its excellent maintenance of a natural breast shape (see Case No. 1).

Case No. 1

A 58-year-old patient underwent a left-breast wide lumpectomy and sentinel node biopsy with positive inferior margins. The patient had always wanted a breast reduction. We recommended re-excision as part of breast reduction.

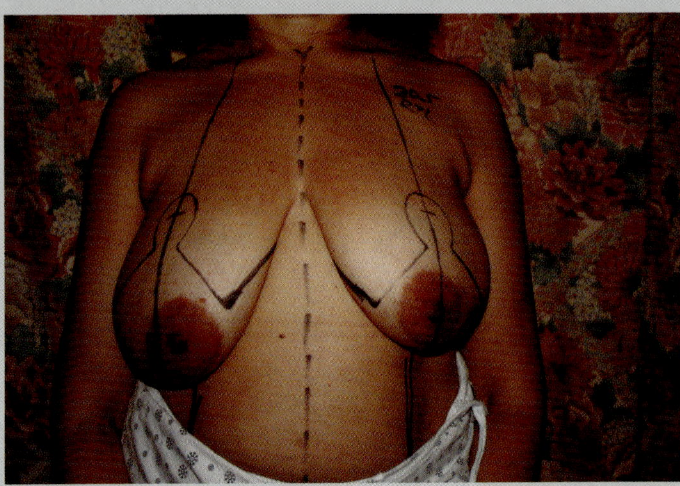

Image 1.1. Preoperative view.

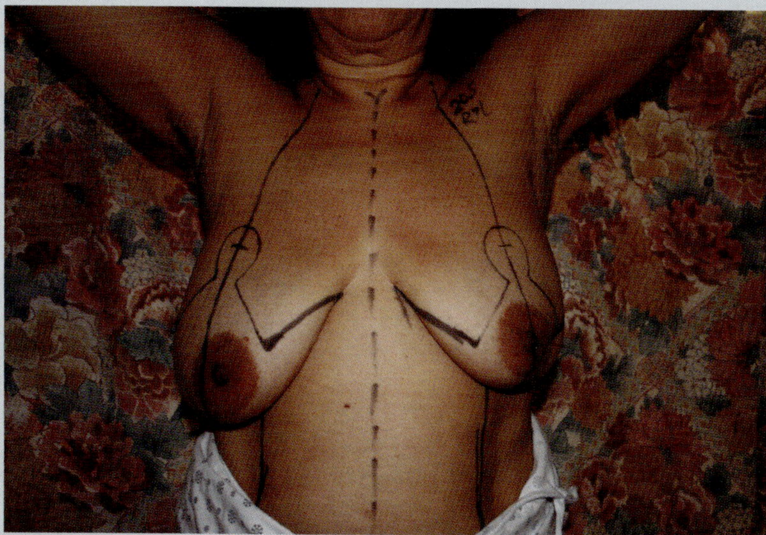

Image 1.2. Preoperative view.

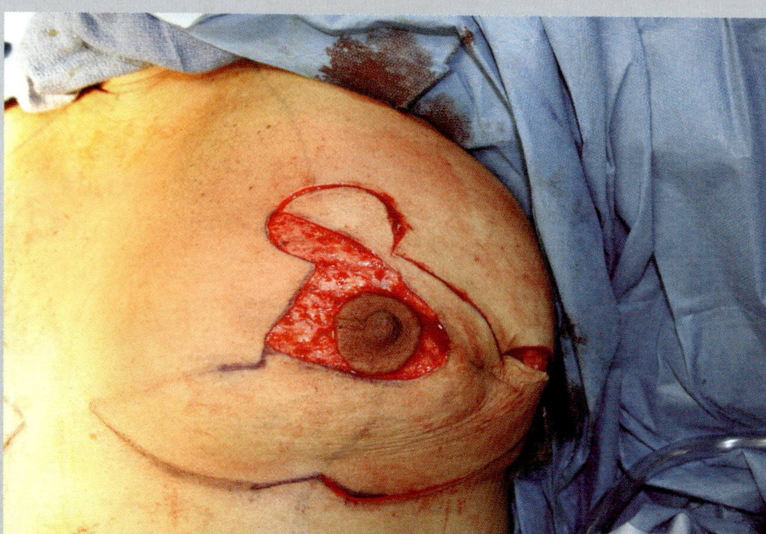

Image 1.3. A superio-medial pedicle was planned as the resection would include the majority of the lower outer quadrant. The skin of the pedicle was de-epithelialized. The rest of the skin seen within the Wise pattern will be excised.

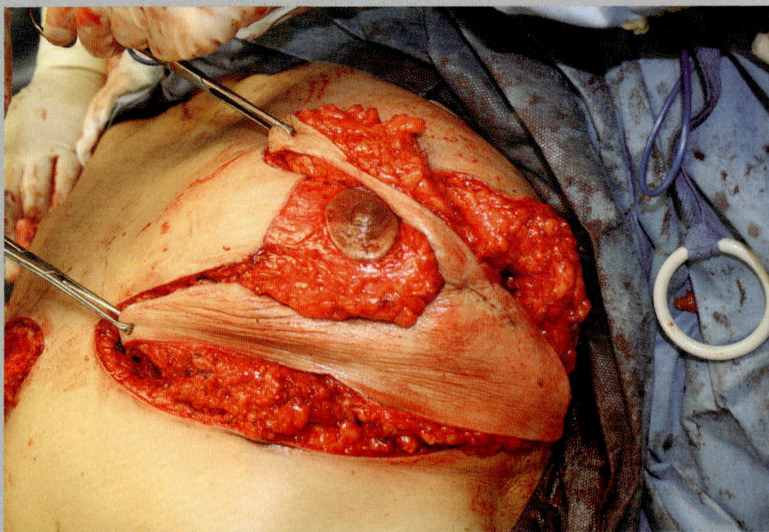

Image 1.4. The resected tissue included the skin and breast tissue within the Wise pattern.

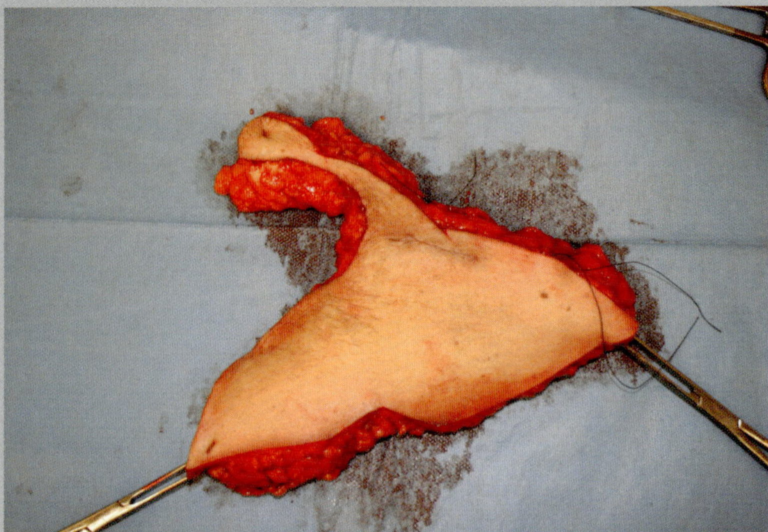

Image 1.5. The specimen of breast skin and resected tissue.

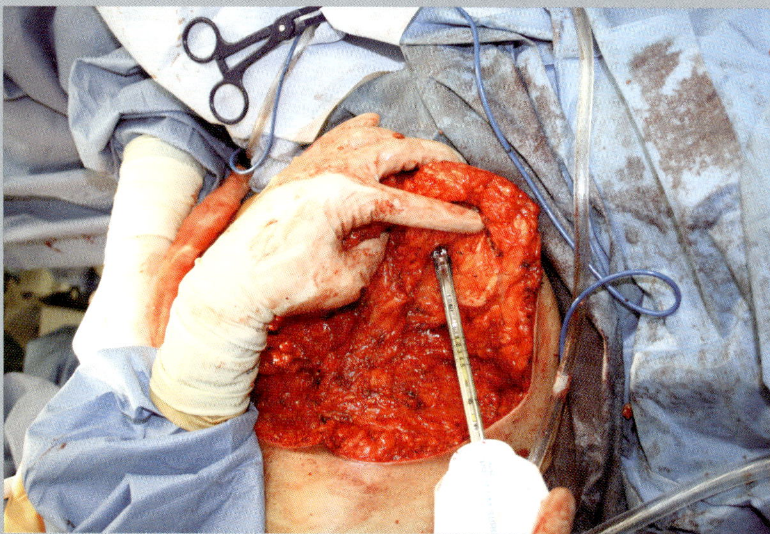

Image 1.6. Metallic clips are applied to mark the margins of resection. They allow the radiation oncologist to boost the lumpectomy bed.

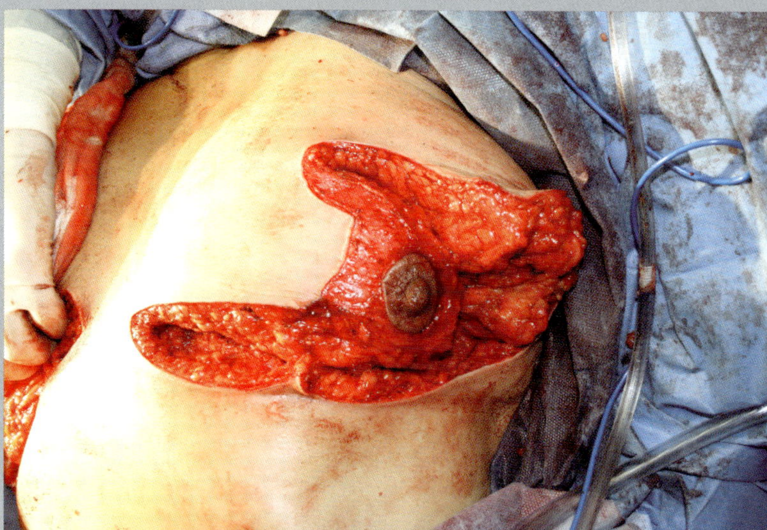

Image 1.7. The final defect, with the nipple based on a superio-medial pedicle for blood supply.

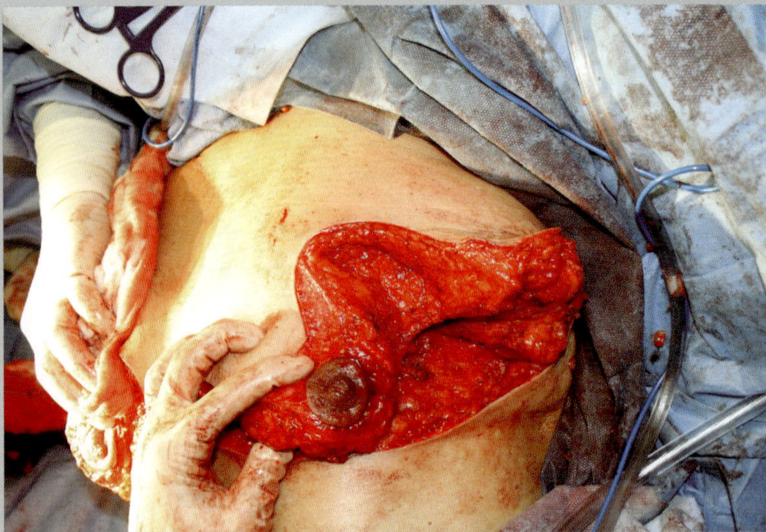

Image 1.8. The NAC pedicle prior to rotation into its new position.

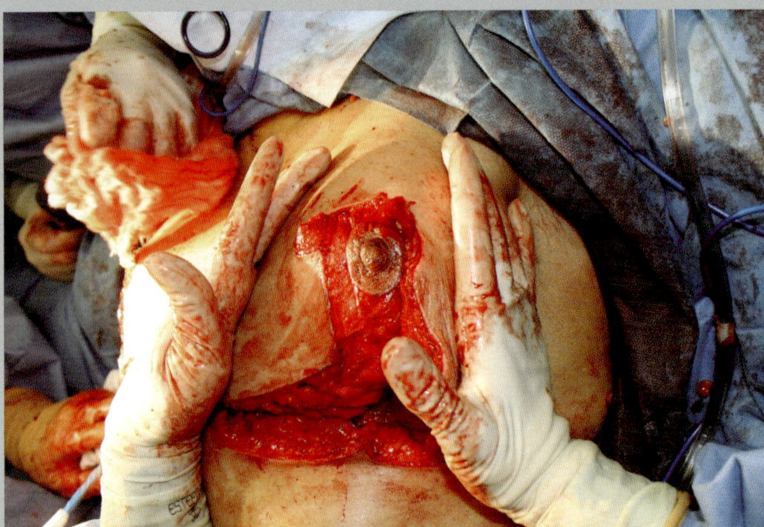

Image 1.9. The NAC rotated into its new position. Notice the 2 vertical limbs of the Wise pattern being approximated.

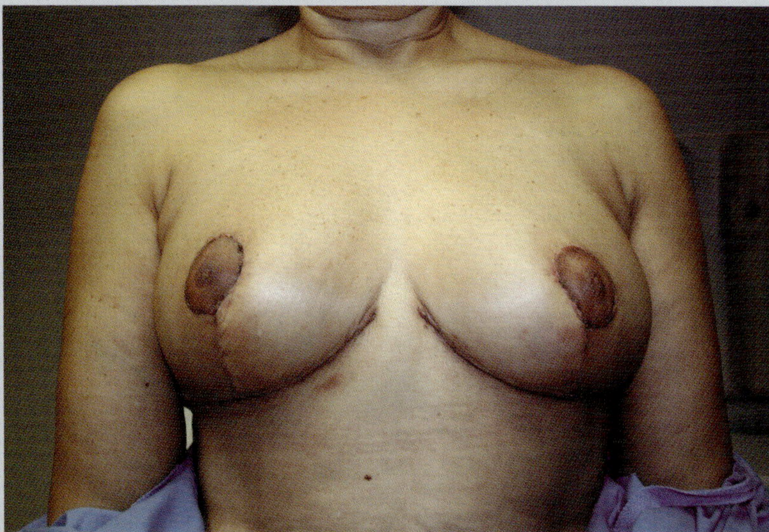

Image 1.10. The patient as seen 2 weeks after surgery. The pathology showed negative margins of resection.

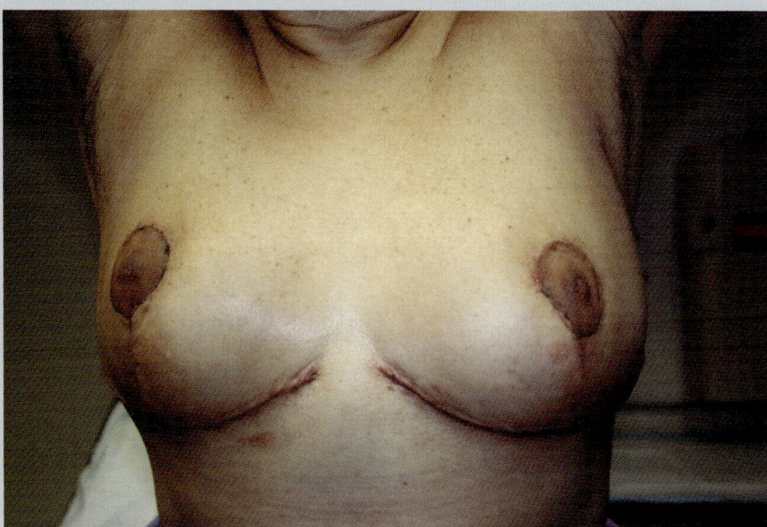

Image 1.11. Postoperative view.

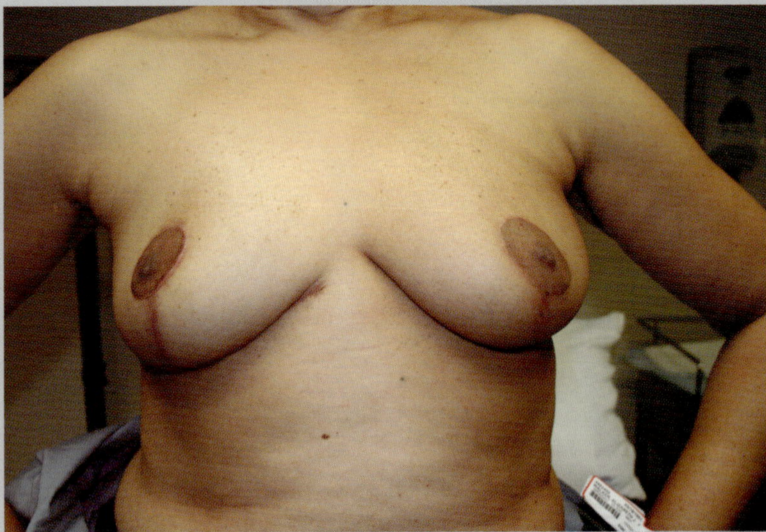

Image 1.12. The patient seen 1 year postoperatively. She had completed all her treatment, including RT.

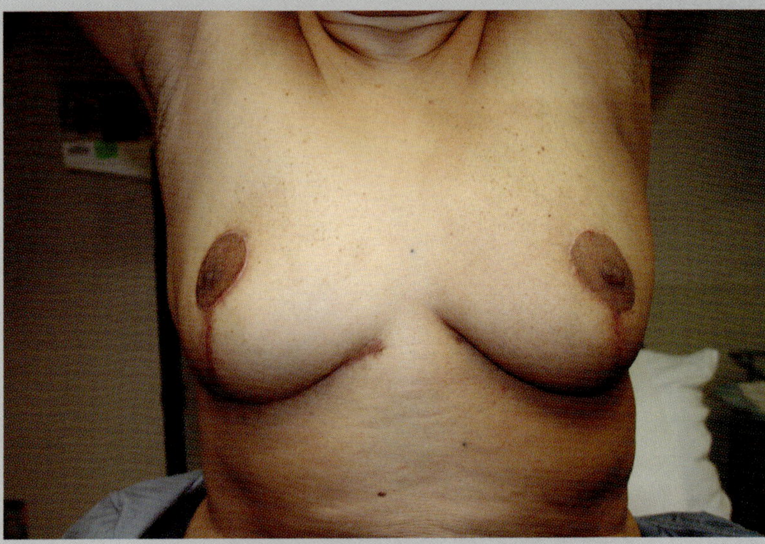

Image 1.13. One year after surgery.

The inferior pedicle technique is very common and reliable. A concern with the inferior pedicle technique, however, is that it lacks parenchymal support and that eventually the breast may sag or "bottom out", which means that there will be excess skin and tissue between the nipple and IMF. While shortening the nipple-IMF distance can help counteract this tendency, it must be balanced against excessively tight closure and the risk of wound-healing complications. This is the pedicle of choice for larger breasts with longer sternal notch-to-nipple distances. The inferior pedicle is a good choice for tumors located in the upper quadrants of the breast (see Case No. 2 for inferior pedicle).

Case No. 2

A 42-year-old patient presented to the plastic surgeons for breast reduction. The surgeon palpated 2 masses in the right breast and 1 in the left. We performed a needle biopsy of all the palpable lesions and identified a 5 cm malignant Cystosarcoma Phyllodes in the upper outer quadrant of the right breast. The 2 other lesions were benign fibroadenomas measuring 3.5 cm each, the first located in the upper inner quadrant of the right breast, and the second in the upper outer quadrant of the left breast.

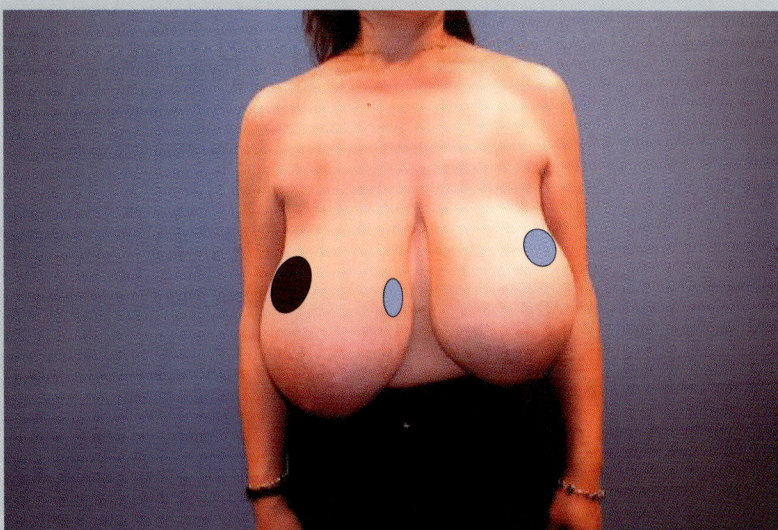

Image 2.1. The patient as seen preoperatively with marking delineating the location of the masses. The dark green mass is the malignant Phyllodes tumor. The light blue masses are the fibroadenomas.

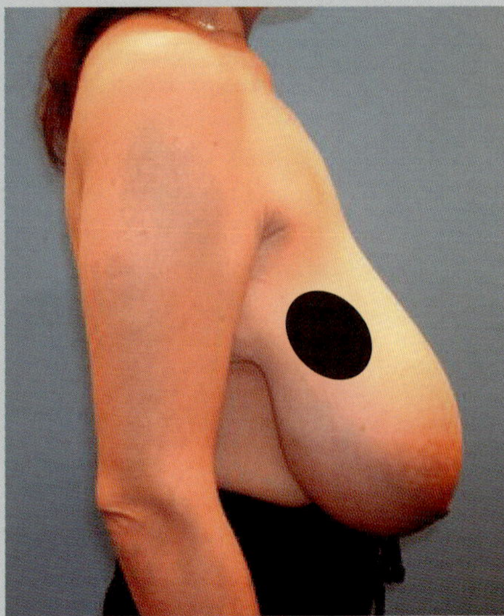

Image 2.2. The lateral view of the right breast in the preoperative period. The dark green mass is the malignant Phyllodes tumor.

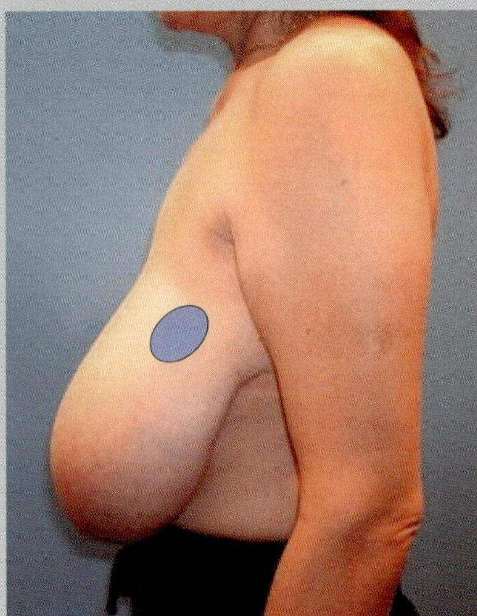

Image 2.3. The lateral view of the left breast in the preoperative period. The light blue mass is one of the fibroadenomas.

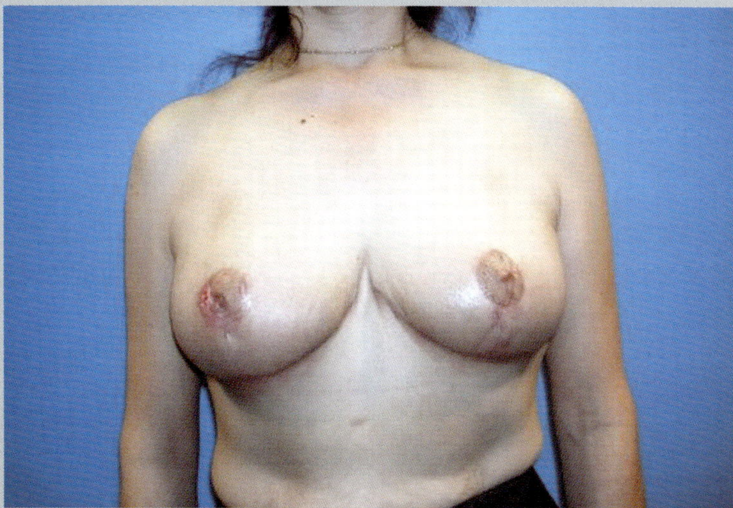

Image 2.4. The patient seen 8 weeks postoperatively. Notice the partial epidermolysis of the lateral aspect of the right nipple and NAC necrosis. To avoid such complications, some surgeons prefer to use a free nipple-areola graft in patients with similarly large and pendulous breasts. We elected to keep the NAC attached to the inferior pedicle.

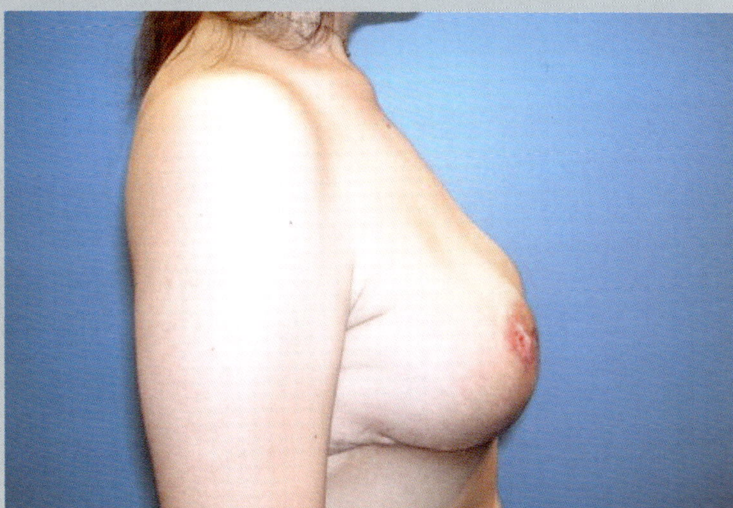

Image 2.5. Lateral view of the right breast in the eighth postoperative week. Again, note the parital epidermolysis of the right areola.

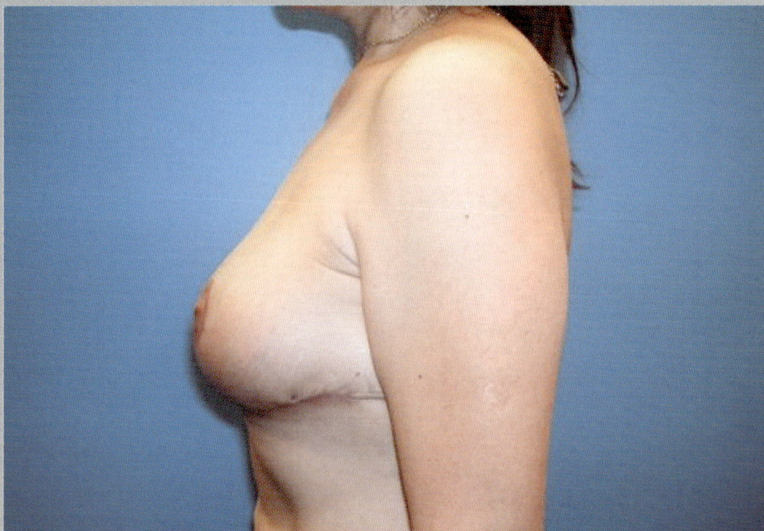

Image 2.6. Lateral view of the left breast in the eighth postoperative week.

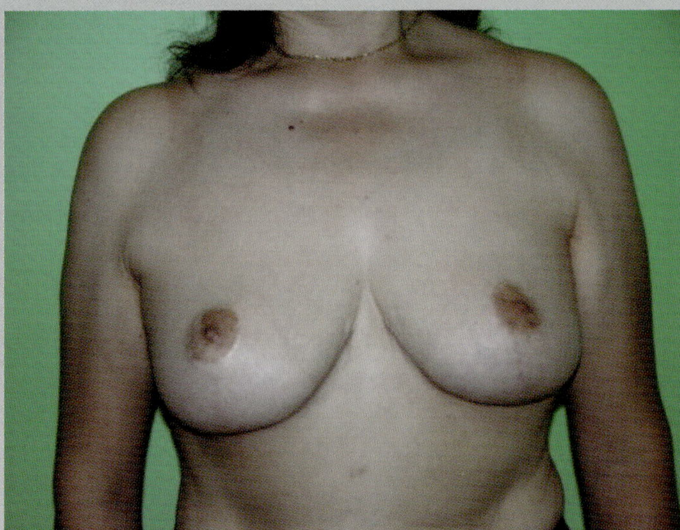

Image 2.7. The patient 2 years after surgery. Notice the complete healing of the right areola. The patient has been doing well 6 years after surgery without any recurrence.

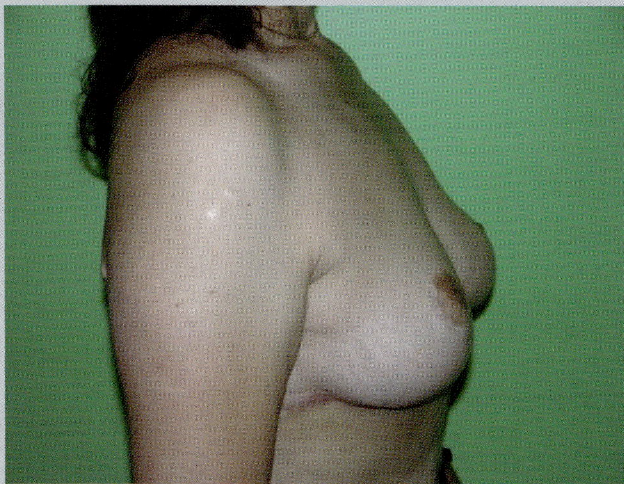

Image 2.8. Lateral view of the right breast showing very good oncologic and cosmetic results 2 years after her procedure.

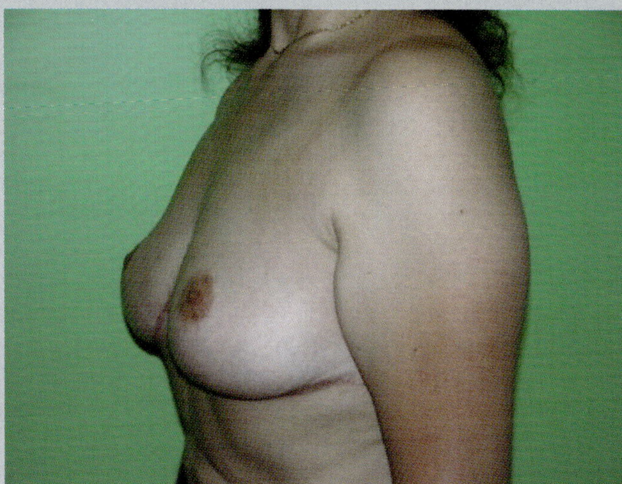

Image 2.9. Lateral view of the left breast 2 years after surgery.

The lateral pedicle may be necessary for medially located tumors which extend into the upper or lower quadrants. The main problem with this pedicle and the reason it is not often used in cosmetic surgery is the resultant lateral fullness of the breast if the pedicle is too thick. This is normally only a technique for women with small-to-moderate–sized breasts who require a mastopexy or a minor reduction.

In women with gigantomastia, attempts to preserve the blood supply and nerves to the nipple during reduction mammaplasty are limited by the length of the pedicle needed to carry the NAC into its new position and by the ability to adequately reduce the breast with a large pedicle. These patients are candidates for free-nipple grafting.

Losken *et al.* demonstrated the ability to use either superomedial or inferior pedicles for tumors in almost any position. Because the most common location for breast cancers is the upper outer quadrant, the most commonly used pedicle was the superomedial.[16] Munhoz *et al.* recommended superior pedicles in almost all tumors except for superior pole tumors. In those patients, he recommended an inferior pedicle.[34] Most recently, Kronowitz *et al.* from the University of Texas MD Anderson Cancer Center divided the breast into 7 zones composed of the 4 quadrants, the retroareolar tissue, and the intersection of the upper and lower quadrants on each side. They proposed a guide of pedicles and modifications to achieve local tissue rearrangement by transposing the NAC, as well as filling the tissue defect.[35]

## 8.10 Radiation Therapy

The second phase of BCT consists of breast irradiation. RT is generally initiated 4 to 6 weeks after the reduction procedure. It consists of whole-breast irradiation, as well as a boost to the tumor bed. The purpose is to clear any remaining microscopic deposit of cells that surgery may have left behind. Aesthetically speaking, an added benefit is that radiation tends to improve the appearance of scars on the breast.[36] In anticipation of radiation, at the time of surgery, attention is directed to avoiding extensive skin-gland dissection and excessively long parenchymal pedicles that may be compromised at this time and predisposed to steatonecrosis.

A concern with oncoplastic breast reduction is the altered topography of the breast parenchyma and not knowing where the true margins of the resection cavity lie. As previously stated, we recommend that the breast surgeons place titanium clips at the edges of the resection to help identify the area for planning of RT and future screening purposes. However, inherent in the breast reduction procedure is complete rearrangement of the local tissues within the breast. With the changed landscape of the breast, the margins of the ablation cavity are shifted and patterns of recurrence altered. For this reason, a mastectomy is most likely indicated if positive margins are identified on final pathology following an oncoplastic breast reduction. In addition, the added boost to the tumor bed, which is the standard treatment, may be compromised as the "cavity", even if marked with clips, no longer exists in the 3-dimensional space it once did.

To correct size asymmetries following RT, it is easier to reduce the contralateral non-irradiated breast than it is to manipulate the radiated breast. It is for the reason of radiation-induced fibrosis and involution that the breast about to undergo radiation is sometimes left slightly larger at the initial surgery. However, with the combination of involution and edema, it is very difficult to estimate the final size of the reconstructed breast. As mentioned earlier, it is for this reason that some surgeons prefer to perform the contralateral symmetrizing reduction in a delayed fashion.

The use of partial-breast irradiation in these cases is limited to intra-operative radiation, brachytherapy, or external beam. The use of balloon radiation is not feasible, as the procedure necessitates closure of the defect and avoidance of seroma. Furthermore, due to the extent of resection with such procedures, the current available balloon size may not allow adequate conformity to the area of resection.

## 8.11 Complications

The complication rate in the literature for oncoplastic bilateral breast reduction ranges from 17% to 24%.[16,34,35] This is significant and a reason why detailed preoperative counseling is so important. The most commonly seen complications are skin necrosis, infection, partial or complete NAC necrosis (Case No. 2, Image 2.4), and suture-line dehiscence. Similar to patients without cancer, those who are obese and regular smokers at the time of surgery suffer from higher complication rates.

It is important to note that most morbidities do not cause a delay in adjuvant treatment. Chemotherapy may not be deterred with a minor complication. However, any complication which does interfere with wound healing may delay the beginning of radiation.

## 8.12 Long-Term Oncologic Results

Up to 4.5 years follow-up, local recurrence varies from 0.0–1.8% per year, while cosmetic dissatisfaction rates vary from 0.0–18.% overall. In the largest study to date, Fitoussi *et al.* followed 540 consecutive patients who underwent primary oncoplastic breast surgery for cancer. All women had high tumor-to-breast–volume ratios and locations which precluded a good aesthetic result with only tumor excision. Techniques included all types of reductions. The median age was 52 years, and median follow-up was

49 months. Average tumor size was 2.9 cm, and most patients started with a B or C brassiere cup size. The mean resection weight was 187 g. Close or involved margins occurred in 18.9%, with mastectomy being necessary in 9.4%. A satisfactory aesthetic outcome at 5 years was obtained in 90.3%. Five-year overall and distant disease-free survival rates were 92.9% and 87.9%, respectively, with local recurrence in 6.8%.[19] These results are comparable to standard BCT, demonstrating the equivalent oncologic safety of the oncoplastic approach.

Caruso *et al.* identified 63 breast cancers in 61 patients, with a median age of 45 years, which were suitable for conservation. All but 1 patient had tumors smaller than 5 cm. All patients were treated with bilateral breast reductions. Tumors in the inferior pole of the breast were treated with the superior pedicle technique. Lesions in the upper pole, inferolateral, or inferomedial were removed with an inferior pedicle reduction. Breasts that were of small and medium size required a periareolar approach, regardless of cancer location. Negative margin was defined as 2 mm between tumor and edge of specimen. All patients underwent whole-breast irradiation with a boost to the tumor bed postoperatively. At a mean follow-up of 68 months, 56 patients were alive. One patient recurred locally, but remained alive and free of disease. She was initially diagnosed with an invasive lobular cancer, which can prove challenging on pathologic analysis. Five developed distant recurrences, of whom only 1 survived.[38] These data demonstrate the safety of the oncoplastic approach, but highlight the challenge of dealing with invasive lobular cancer, which has more insidious margins than its ductal counterpart.

Rietjens *et al.*, in a series of 148 cases with a median follow-up of 74 months, reported a 3% rate of local recurrence.[38] The authors did not observe any local recurrence for lesions below 2 cm. Kayar *et al.* reported a series of 116 patients in which the mean specimen weight was 659 g per side. The 10-year overall survival rate was 100% for stage I, 89.1% for stage II, and 53.8% for stage III.[39]

## 8.13 Breast Cancer Surveillance

Complex glandular reshaping could become a challenge for less-experienced breast radiotherapists and for breast radiologists dealing with follow-up mammograms. In 2009, Losken *et al.* evaluated long-term postoperative breast cancer surveillance in women who had undergone partial breast reconstruction. Seventeen patients with an average follow-up of 6.3 years were retrospectively reviewed and compared to 17 women who had undergone BCT alone. Mammographic findings, such as architectural distortion, cysts, and calcifications were similar between the 2 groups. No significant difference existed in breast density. The women with oncoplastic reductions had longer times to mammographic stabilization (21.2 months versus 25.6 months); however, this was not clinically significant. An expected trend toward a greater number of postoperative mammograms and ultrasounds was found in the study group. In addition, the rate of tissue sampling in the study group was significantly higher (53%) versus that of the control group (18%).[40]

The ability to screen for cancer recurrence does not seem to be affected by oncoplastic breast reduction. Scar tissue may appear suspicious on physical exam, mammogram, ultrasound, or MRI. It can be evaluated with fine needle aspiration or, preferably, core needle biopsy. When the oncologic surgeon is clinically uncomfortable with a specific area in the breast, even after extensive imaging and tissue sampling, we do recommend an excisional biopsy for confirmation. Patients may present with fat necrosis that may be suspicious for tumor recurrence. Fat necrosis usually presents early postoperatively, and tends to slowly resolve with time. Resorption of fat necrosis is a slow process and may not be complete. Adequate clinical follow-up by the same oncologic surgeon is important. Mammographic findings after oncoplastic surgery include scarring and fibrosis in 50% of patients, fluid accumulations in 40% of patients, and dystrophic calcifications in 10% of patients.[41] After breast reduction, it is common to see epidermal inclusion cysts or areas of fat necrosis. These can reliably be diagnosed with fine needle aspiration biopsy[42] or core needle biopsies. Losken *et al.* noted that although cancer screening was not compromised, 26% of the patients in his study required some type of postoperative tissue sampling; this number is higher than what is seen in traditional BCT.

## 8.14 Cosmetic and Functional Outcomes

An objective and comparable method for the measurement of cosmetic outcome has been lacking. With the development of the new BREAST-Q, which quantifies patient satisfaction and health-related quality of life experienced by women undergoing breast reconstruction, this may change. But for now, generally speaking, the published literature and our personal experiences demonstrate uniformly satisfied patients. Chang *et al.* evaluated the degree of patient satisfaction with cosmetic form and function via a survey of 37 patients. Twenty of the 37 responded, with 70% rating the cosmetic outcome as excellent. All responders expressed a high degree of satisfaction with cosmetic and functional results, and stated that they would choose this technique if they had to undergo cancer surgery again.[43] Goffman *et al.*

published a study of 55 patients evaluated by a panel, including a surgical oncologist, an oncology nurse, a radiation oncologist, and a patient, with 72% of the evaluations reporting "excellent" and "very good" results.[44] Losken *et al.* noted that 95% of women defined their aesthetic result as satisfactory at their 6-month follow-up exams.[16]

## 8.15 Future Directions

Breast surgeons are becoming increasingly interested in performing the reconstructive portion of the operation, as well as the ablative portion. There are numerous reasons for this shift. In some places in the United States, there may be a potential lack of willing and available reconstructive plastic surgeons. Coordination of the combined surgeon approach can also pose scheduling difficulties. Breast surgeons are then motivated to either perform both components of the surgery, or to send the patient to a large referral center for the combined procedure.[45]

Management of the patient with breast cancer is changing. Even though breast cancer has not been eradicated through research, those who treat breast cancer patients are constantly striving for less-invasive and more aesthetically pleasing ways to help patients manage this disease and live with the aftereffects of their treatment. As physicians treating breast cancer, we have come a long way since the time of the Halsted radical mastectomy, but there is still much progress to be made. As plastic surgeons in the multidisciplinary breast cancer team, our expertise places us in a prime spot to be a part of that progress and to maintain an active involvement in the future progression of breast cancer treatment.

## References

1. Canady JW, D'Amico RA, McGuire MF. (2009) Discussion. Oncoplastic breast surgery: Past, present, and future directions in the United States. *Plast Reconstr Surg* 124(3):973–974.
2. Fisher B, Anderson S, Bryant J, *et al.* (2002) Twenty-year follow-up of a randomized trial comparing total mastectomy, lumpectomy, and lumpectomy plus irradiation for the treatment of invasive breast cancer. *N Engl J Med* 347(16):1233–1241.
3. Clough KB, Cuminet J, Fitoussi A, *et al.* (1998) Cosmetic sequelae after conservative treatment for breast cancer: Classification and results of surgical correction. *Ann Plast Surg* 41(5):471–481.
4. D'Aniello C, Grimaldi L, Barbato A, *et al.* (1999) Cosmetic results in 242 patients treated by conservative surgery for breast cancer. *Scand J Plast Reconstr Surg Hand Surg* 33(4):419–422.

5. Petit JY, Rietjens M, Garusi C, *et al.* (1998) Integration of plastic surgery in the course of breast-conserving surgery for cancer to improve cosmetic results and radicality of tumor excision. *Recent Results Cancer Res* 152:202–211.
6. Clough KB, Soussaline M, Campana F, Salmon RJ. (1990) Mammoplasty combined with irradiation: Conservative treatment of breast cancer localized in the lower quadrant. *Ann Chir Plast Aesthet* 35(2):117–122.
7. Audretsch W, Rezai M, Kolotas C. (1998) Tumor-specific immediate reconstruction in breast cancer patients. *Perspect Plast Surg* 11:71–100.
8. Munhoz AM, Montag E, Arruda E, *et al.* (2008) Assessment of immediate conservative breast surgery reconstruction: A classification system of defects revisited and an algorithm for selecting the appropriate technique. *Plast Reconstr Surg* 121(3):716–727.
9. Kaur N, Petit JY, Rietjens M, *et al.* (2005) Comparative study of surgical margins in oncoplastic surgery and quadrantectomy in breast cancer. *Ann Surg Oncol* 12(7):539–545.
10. Cochrane RA, Valasiadou P, Wilson AR, *et al.* (2003) Cosmesis and satisfaction after breast-conserving surgery correlates with the percentage of breast volume excised. *Br J Surg* 90(12):1505–1509.
11. Clough KB. (2008) Keynote speech: Oncoplastic surgery. Presented at the RACS/CSHK Conjoint Annual Scientific Congress, Hong Kong, May.
12. Dundas KL, Atyeo J, Cox J. (2007) What is a large breast? Measuring and categorizing breast size for tangential breast radiation therapy. *Australas Radiol* 51(6):589–593.
13. Taylor ME, Perez CA, Halverson KJ, *et al.* (1995) Factors influencing cosmetic results after conservation therapy for breast cancer. *Int J Radiat Oncol Biol Phys* 31(4):753–764.
14. Hernanz F, Regano S, Vega A, Gomez Fleitas M. (2009) Reduction mammaplasty: An advantageous option for breast conserving surgery in large-breasted patients. *Surg Oncol* 19(4):e95–e102.
15. Rietjens M, Petit JY, Contesso G. (1997) The role of reduction mammaplasty in oncology. *Eur J Plast Surg* 20(5):246–249.
16. Losken A, Styblo TM, Carlson GW, *et al.* (2007) Management algorithm and outcome evaluation of partial mastectomy defects treated using reduction or mastopexy techniques. *Ann Plast Surg* 59(3):235–242.
17. Dieffenbach JF. (1848) *Die Operative Chirurgie,* Vol 2. Brockhaus, Leipzig.
18. Adams WP. (2002) Reduction mammaplasty and mastopexy. *Select Read Plast Surg* 9(29):5.
19. Fitoussi AD, Berry MG, Fama F, *et al.* (2010) Oncoplastic breast surgery for cancer: Analysis of 540 consecutive cases [outcomes article]. *Plast Reconstr Surg* 125(2):454–462.
20. Penn J. (1955) Breast reduction. *Br J Plast Surg* 7(4):357–371.
21. Schnitt SJ. (2003) Risk factors for local recurrence in patients with invasive breast cancer and negative surgical margins of excision. Where are we and where are we going? *Am J Clin Pathol* 120(4):485–488.
22. Singletary SE. (2002) Surgical margins in patients with early-stage breast cancer treated with breast conservation therapy. *Am J Surg* 184(5):383–393.

23. Haid A, Knauer M, Dunzinger S, *et al.* (2007) Intra-operative sonography: A valuable aid during breast-conserving surgery for occult breast cancer. *Ann Surg Oncol* 14(11):3090–3101.
24. Rahusen FD, Bremers AJ, Fabry HF, *et al.* (2002) Ultrasound-guided lumpectomy of nonpalpable breast cancer versus wire-guided resection: A randomized clinical trial. *Ann Surg Oncol* 9(10):994–998.
25. Pappo I, Spector R, Schindel A, *et al.* (2010) Diagnostic performance of a novel device for real-time margin assessment in lumpectomy specimens. *J Surg Res* 160(2):277–281.
26. Pleijhuis RG, Graafland M, de Vries J, *et al.* (2009) Obtaining adequate surgical margins in breast-conserving therapy for patients with early-stage breast cancer: Current modalities and future directions. *Ann Surg Oncol* 16(10):2717–2730.
27. Silverstein MJ, Lagios MD, Groshen S, *et al.* (1999) The influence of margin width on local control of ductal carcinoma *in situ* of the breast. *N Engl J Med* 340(19):1455–1461.
28. Lassus C. (1987) Breast reduction: Evolution of a technique – A single vertical scar. *Aesthet Plast Surg* 11(2):107–112.
29. Lejour M. (1994) Vertical mammaplasty and liposuction of the breast. *Plast Reconstr Surg* 94(1):100–114.
30. Benelli L. (1990) A new periareolar mammaplasty: The "round block" technique. *Aesthet Plast Surg* 14(2):93–100.
31. Berry MG, Ballester M, Fitoussi A, *et al.* (2008) Lateral mammaplasty for oncoplastic breast surgery. *Eur J Surg Oncol* 34:1156.
32. Anderson BO, Masetti R, Silverstein MJ. (2005) Oncoplastic approaches to partial mastectomy: An overview of volume-displacement techniques. *Lancet Oncol* 6(3):145–157.
33. Strauch B, Elkowitz M, Baum T, Herman C. (2005) Superolateral pedicle for breast surgery: An operation for all reasons. *Plast Reconstr Surg* 115(5):1269–1277; discussion 78–79.
34. Munhoz AM, Montag E, Arruda EG, *et al.* (2006) Critical analysis of reduction mammaplasty techniques in combination with conservative breast surgery for early breast cancer treatment. *Plast Reconstr Surg* 117(4):1091–1103; discussion 104–107.
35. Kronowitz SJ, Hunt KK, Kuerer HM, *et al.* (2007) Practical guidelines for repair of partial mastectomy defects using the breast reduction technique in patients undergoing breast conservation therapy. *Plast Reconstr Surg* 120(7):1755–1768.
36. Clough KB, Nos C, Salmon RJ, *et al.* (1995) Conservative treatment of breast cancers by mammaplasty and irradiation: A new approach to lower quadrant tumors. *Plast Reconstr Surg* 96(2):363–370.
37. Caruso F, Catanuto G, De Meo L, *et al.* (2008) Outcomes of bilateral mammoplasty for early stage breast cancer. *Eur J Surg Oncol* 34(10):1143–1147.
38. Rietjens M, Urban CA, Rey PC, *et al.* (2007) Long-term oncological results of breast conservative treatment with oncoplastic surgery. *Breast* 16(4):387–395.

39. Kayar R, Cobanoglu M, Gungor O, *et al.* (2006) The value of breast reduction operations in breast conservation surgery; late results of 116 patients with breast cancer. *Meme Sagligi Dergisi* 2:131–138.
40. Losken A, Schaefer TG, Newell M, Styblo TM. (2009) The impact of partial breast reconstruction using reduction techniques on postoperative cancer surveillance. *Plast Reconstr Surg* 124(1):9–17.
41. Mendelsohn AM, Bove EL, Lupinetti FM, *et al.* (1994) Central pulmonary artery growth patterns after the bidirectional Glenn procedure. *J Thorac Cardiovasc Surg* 107(5):1284–1290.
42. Fajardo LL, Bessen SC. (1993) Epidermal inclusion cyst after reduction mammoplasty. *Radiology* 186(1):103–106.
43. Chang E, Johnson N, Webber B, *et al.* (2004) Bilateral reduction mammoplasty in combination with lumpectomy for treatment of breast cancer in patients with macromastia. *Am J Surg* 187(5):647–650; discussion 50–51.
44. Goffman TE, Schneider H, Hay K, *et al.* (2005) Cosmesis with bilateral mammoreduction for conservative breast cancer treatment. *Breast J* 11(3):195–198.
45. Losken A, Nahabedian MY. (2009) Oncoplastic breast surgery: Past, present, and future directions in the United States. *Plast Reconstr Surg* 124(3):969–972.

# Chapter 9

# MASTOPEXY

Mahmoud El-Tamer

*Breast Service, Department of Surgery,*
*Memorial Sloan-Kettering Cancer Center,*
*New York, NY 10065, USA*

## 9.1 Introduction

In patients with a ptotic breast, one can combine a mastopexy (breast lift) to the resection of the tumor. In such procedures, the breast tissue resection is limited to the oncologic procedure only, while the skin incision has a dual purpose:

1. Exposure for resection of the tumor.
2. Resection of the redundant skin in order to tighten the envelope of the breast.

These procedures require mobilization of the nipple areola complex in an upward fashion. We recommend reviewing the text of Chapter 2 for nipple line guidance. These procedures can be extremely gratifying to the patient provided the nipple areola complex remains along the nipple line. Any misplacement of the nipple areola complex, however, will result in a poor cosmetic result that may be quite challenging to repair, particularly after radiation therapy.

In this chapter, we will describe 2 different mastopexy techniques, and variations of those techniques, that allow the oncoplastic surgeon to achieve those goals.

## 9.2 Dome Mastopexy

The dome mastopexy is a very versatile and easy procedure to learn. It allows easy access to central and upper hemisphere tumors. The basis of this procedure is to resect a semicircular ellipse of skin above the areola (Figure 9.1). The lower aspect of the ellipse of the skin incision to be excised extends from the 3 o′clock position to the 9 o′clock position at the upper edge of the areola. The width of the ellipse will dictate the extent of elevation of the nipple areola complex. We have avoided large resection of the skin above the nipple areola complex and limited the width of the ellipse to 2.5–3.0 cm. Significant elevation of the nipple areola complex without adjustment of the distance between the lower edge of the areola and the inframammary line may result in malpositioning of the nipple areola complex. In patients with significant ptosis of the breast that necessitates a larger ellipse or dome, we recommend using a different type of mastopexy technique.

Dome mastopexy procedures are ideal for lesions in the 12 o′clock axis (Figure 9.2) or for lesions underlying the nipple areola complex (Case 1). The skin resection may be used for the purpose of exposure and is resected separately. Alternatively, the skin may be resected *en bloc* with the tumor in one specimen. The lumpectomy does not necessarily need to follow the shape of the overlying skin.

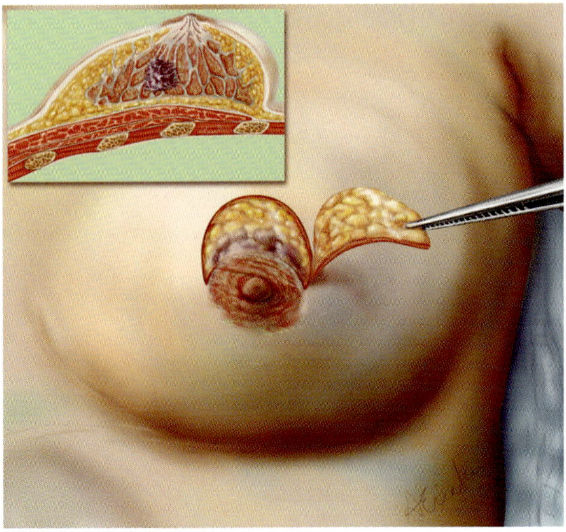

Figure 9.1. Dome incision.

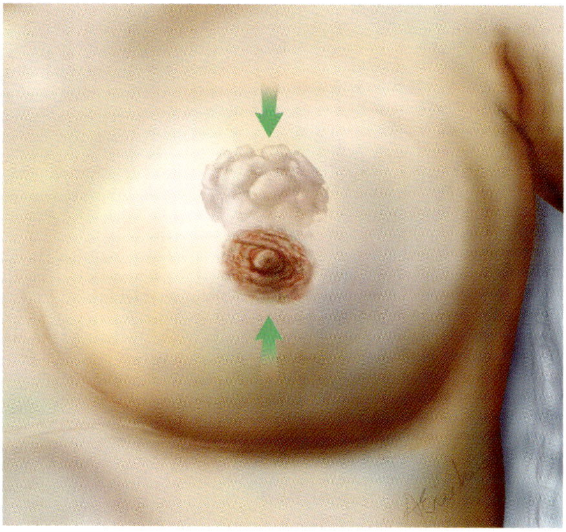

Figure 9.2. Tumors and the ideal location for a dome incision.

Case 1

A 48-year-old woman who presented with 2 breast lesions in the 12 o′clock and subarolar area; both lesions were proven malignant by needle biopsy. The patient was interested in breast conservation. She had a cup size A/B breast with minimal ptosis. The patient wanted to preseve her nipple areola complex. The resection entailed removal of the breast tissue under the nipple arola complex and at the 12 o′clock axis. Repair of the defect after such a large resection resulted in redundancy of the skin, hence the need for partial removal of the overlying skin to be planned in the form of a dome with lateral extension. The width of the dome was minimized to avoid significant elevation of the nipple arola as the patient had minimal ptosis. Following the first resection, the patient had one positive margin that required re-excision.

1. The patient on the operating room table with a wire localizing each tumor. Note the limited width of the dome.
2. The defect following approximation of the deep breast tissue.
3. Skin closure after completion of the repair. Of note, following the first resection, the patient had one positive margin that required re-excision.

4,5. The patient after surgery.

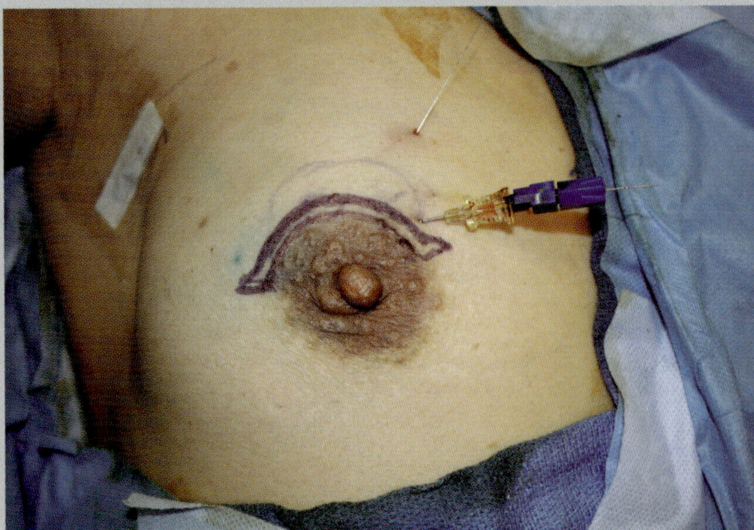

Image 1.1. The patient on the operating room table with a wire localizing each tumor. Note the limited width of the dome.

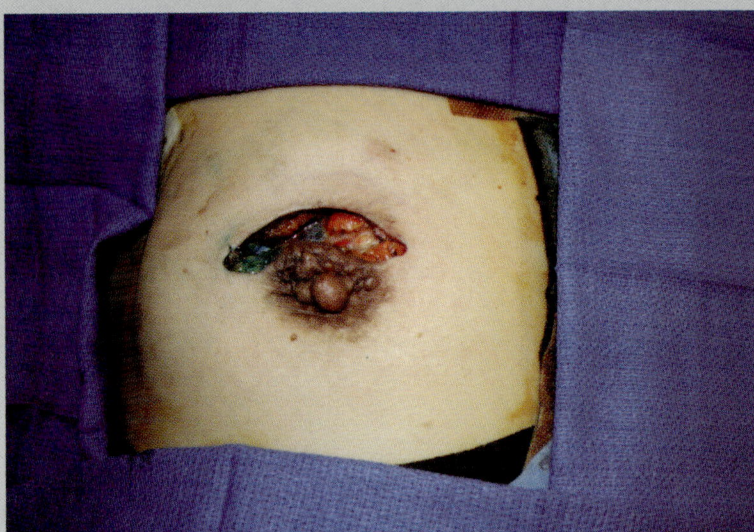

Image 1.2. The defect following approximation of the deep breast tissue.

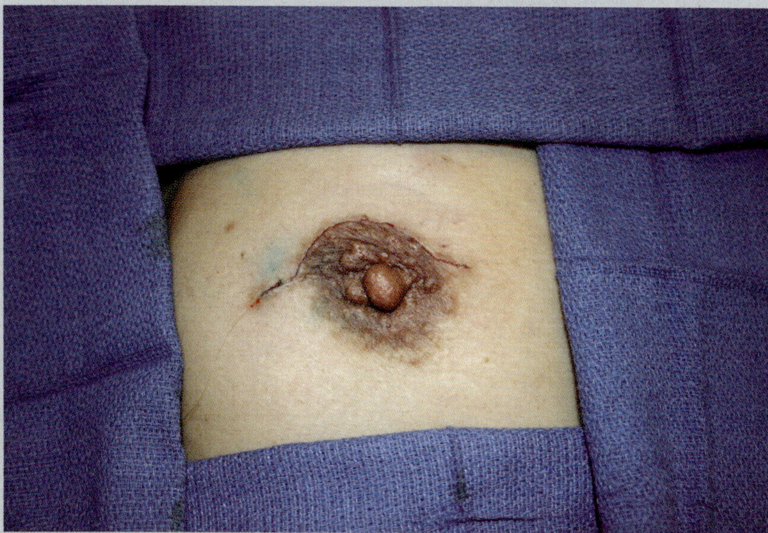

Image 1.3. Skin closure after completion of the repair. Of note, following the first resection, the patient had one positive margin that required re-excision.

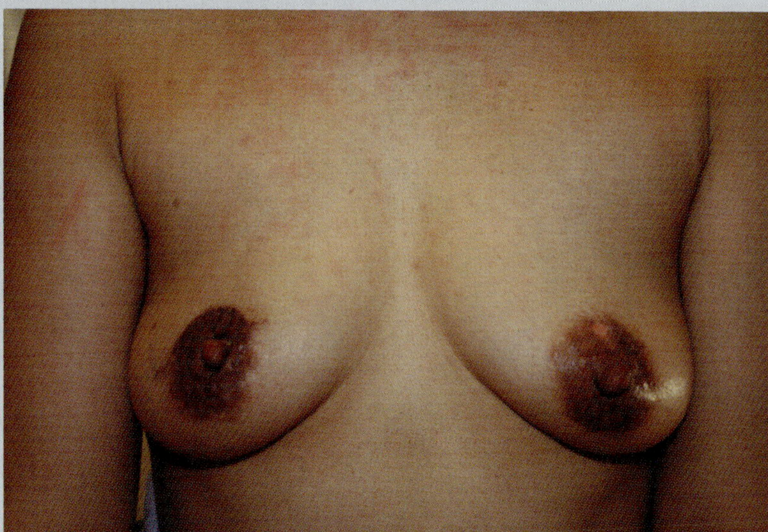

Image 1.4. Patient after surgery.

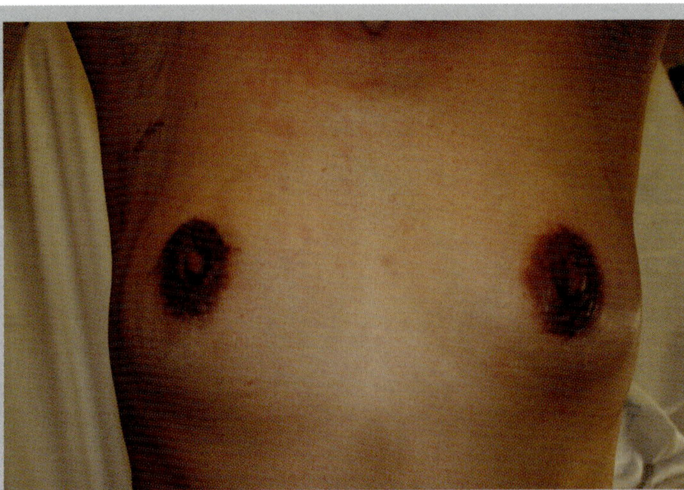

Image 1.5. Patient after surgery.

One of the limiting factors of such an approach is the diameter of the areola. Access to the breast tissue may be limited in patients with small areolas. Due to the nature of blood supply to the nipple areola complex, the maximum length of the ellipse in the dome procedure is limited to 50% of the circumference of the areola; that is equal to the radius of the areola times $\pi$. With a nipple areola complex equal to 2 cm in diameter, the length of the ellipse would be $1 \times \pi = 3.14$ cm. Lateral and/or medial extension may be necessary for patients with small areolas (Figure 9.3).

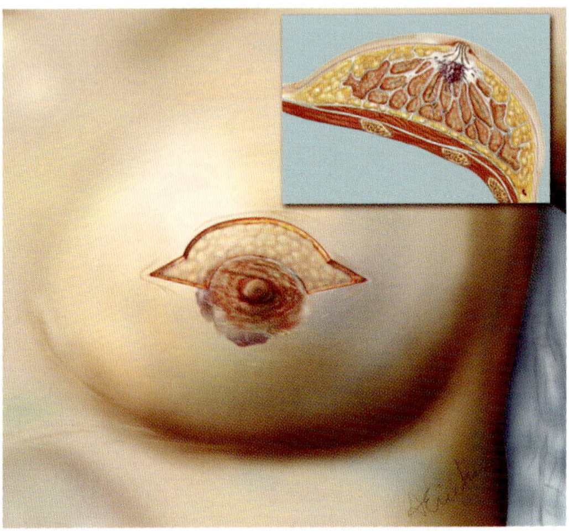

Figure 9.3. Batwing incisions.

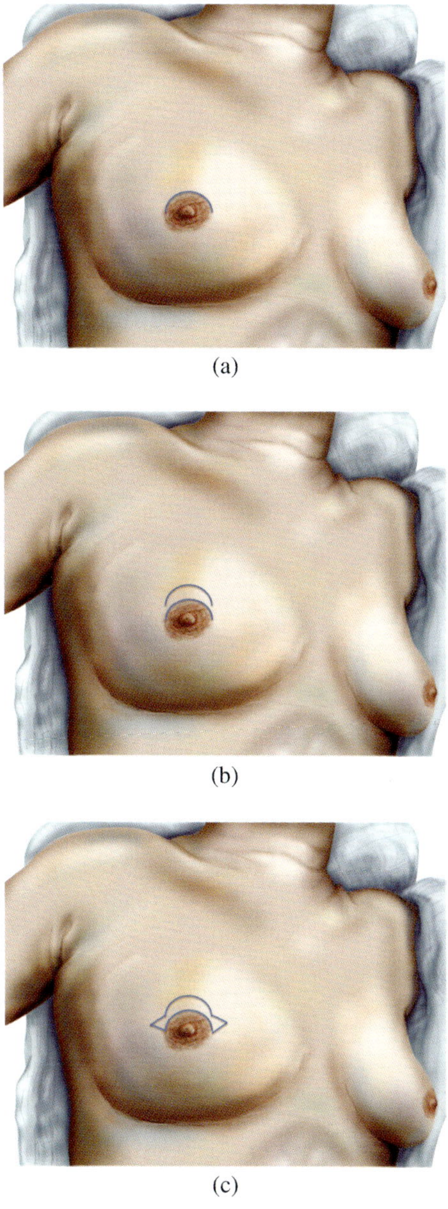

Figure 9.4. Dome with extensions. (a) Draw a semicircle around the upper edge of the areola extending from 3 o′clock to 9 o′clock. (b) Draw exactly the same semicircle at a distance equal to the desired elevation of the nipple. (c) Draw equidistant lines from the edges of the semi-circles. The lengths of these lateral/medial extensions depend on the extent of exposure desired. The wider the exposure, the longer the lines.

The lateral/medial extensions are of a limited distance and serve mainly to enhance exposure. These extensions are in the form of an extra triangle of skin to be excised medially and laterally. Bilateral triangular extensions to the dome have been popularized as "batwings" by Dr. Melvin Silverstein[1] or as the "Omega technique" by the Institut Curie group.[2,3]

The design of a dome with medial and lateral extensions is demonstrated in Figures 9.4a–c. Please refer to Case 1 for a clinical example of a dome mastopexy with a central tumor. Figures 9.5 and 9.6 demonstrate the batwing defect and repair for a subareolar tumor. With the dome incision, it is obvious that the upper edge of the skin incision is longer than the lower or peri-areolar edge.

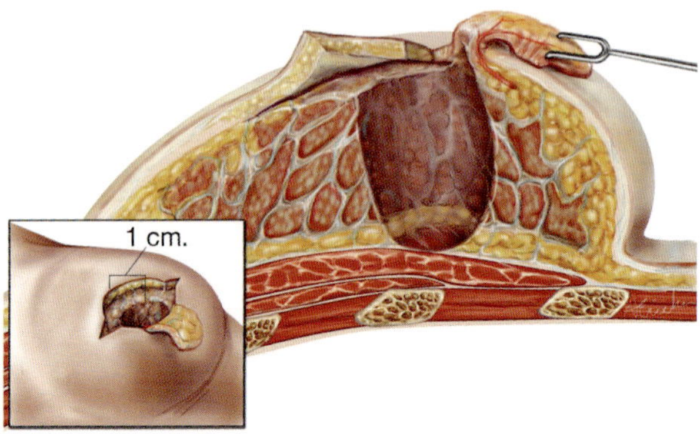


Figure 9.5. "Batwing" or "dome" defect. The width of the dome in this drawing was set at 1 cm. The width is dependent on the desired nipple areola complex elevation.

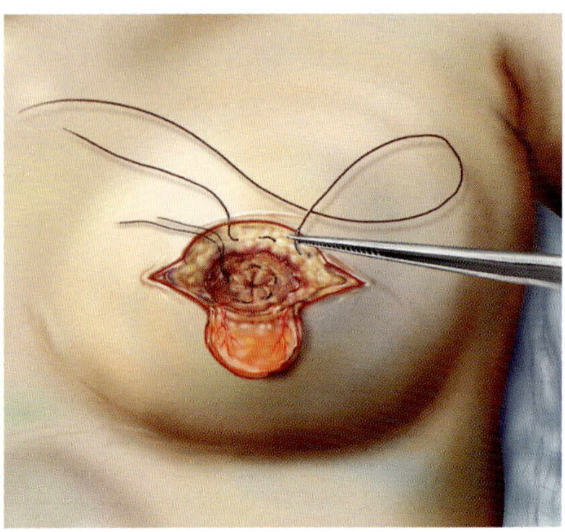

Figure 9.6. Batwing closure.

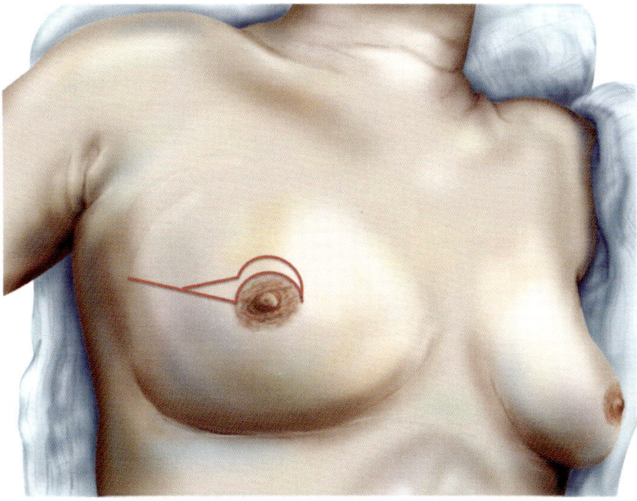

(a)

Figure 9.7. (a) Combining dome mastopexy and radial resection. The main purpose of this radial extension is exposure for a laterally located tumor.

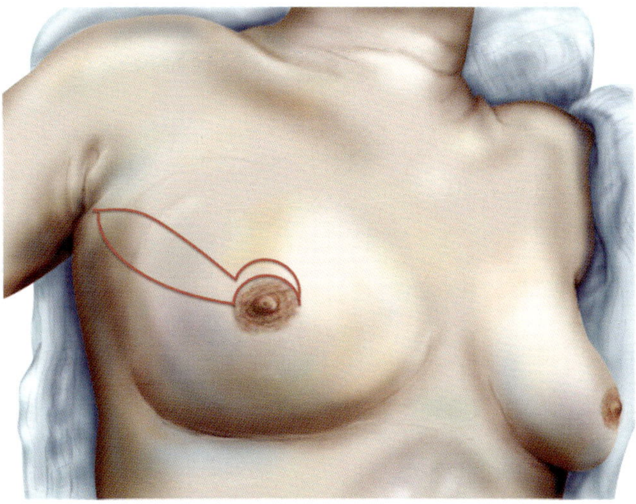

(b)

Figure 9.7. (b) Dome mastopexy with extension to excise an ellipse of skin overlying the tumor. The skin of the dome may be only de-epithelialized as in Case No. 2, Image 2.4. Again, the width of the dome depends on the extent of nipple areola complex elevation desired.

The "dome" technique may be combined with a radial resection. The combination of these 2 techniques allows elevation of the nipple areola complex with resection of a peripheral tumor Figure 9.7(a). The radial resection may be designed to include an *en bloc* excision of the tumor with the overlying skin when indicated as in Figure 9.7(b) and in Case No. 2, Images 2.2 and 2.3. With this combination, we do not recommend full resection of the skin and breast tissue of the dome. We feel that simply removing the epithelial layer of the dome or its skin will be sufficient for achieving the nipple areola elevation while maintaining its neurovascular supply (Case 2, Image 2.4). The dome with unilateral radial extension tumor was popularized as "hemi-batwing" By Dr. Silverstein[4] and described in detail by the Institute Curie group.[5]

Case 2

A 54-year-old woman underwent a large resection of a right breast tumor located in the 3 o′clock axis with positive superior and medial margins. The resection resulted in a deformity of the breast. The plan was to re-excise the positive margins and perform a mastopexy in the same setting.

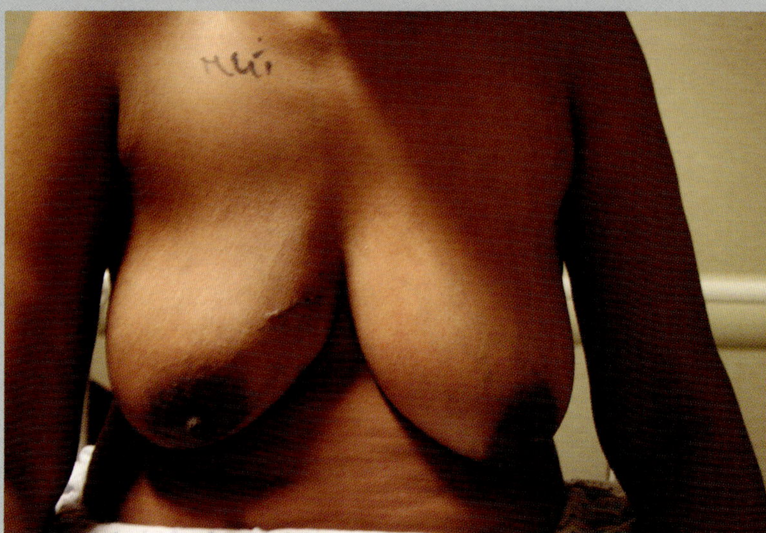

Image 2.1. The patient preoperatively with significant loss of volume in the medial aspect of the right breast associated with deviation of the nipple medially.

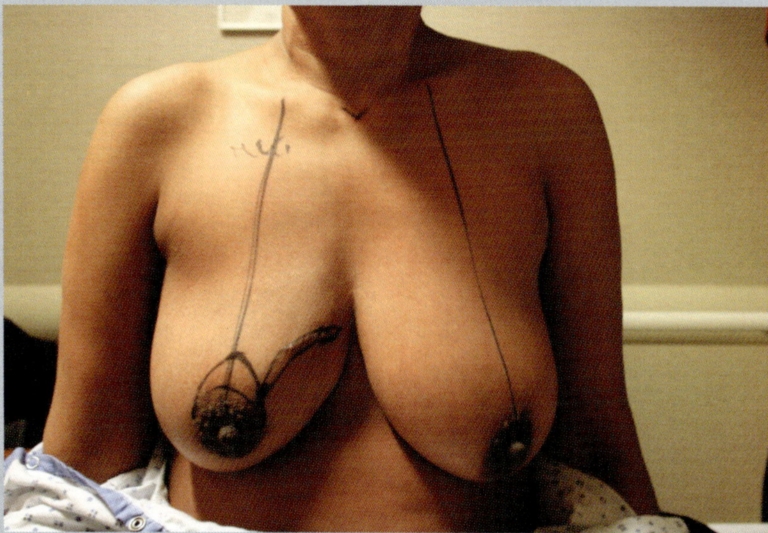

Image 2.2. The nipple line has been marked in the erect position with a preliminary plan of resection and mastopexy.

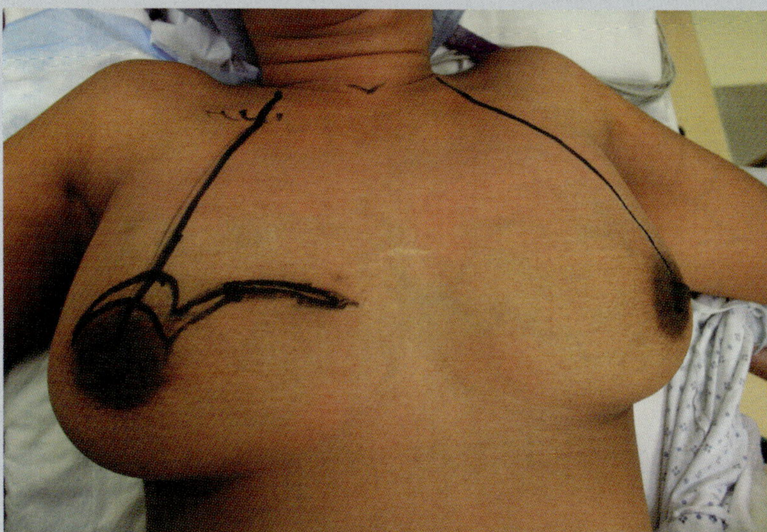

Image 2.3. The patient on the operating table.

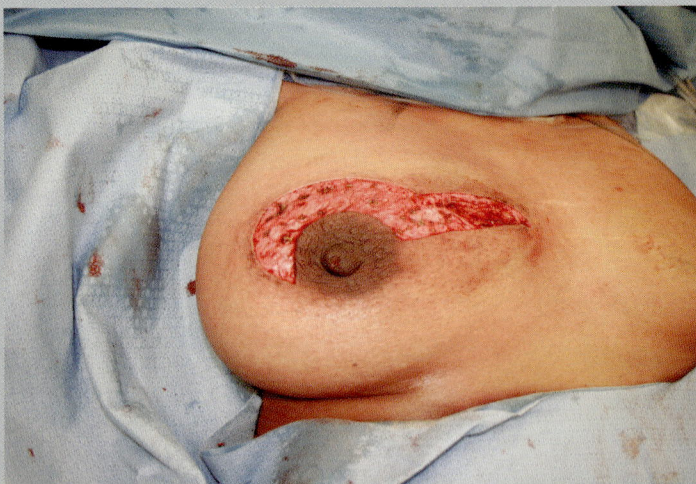

Image 2.4. Following margin resection, the patient was positioned at a 75-degree back-up position; the mastopexy was replanned by stapling the edge of the areola to its new position. It was evident that the extent of skin resection needed to be modified. Note the resection of the skin and margins was performed *en bloc* down to the fascia, whereas the skin over the dome was only de-epithelialized.

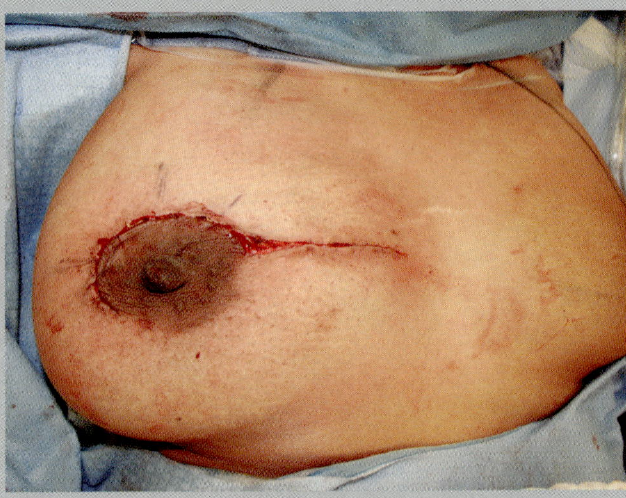

Image 2.5. The skin of the upper edge of the dome was elevated off the breast to a 1-cm distance. The edge of the areola was approximated to the upper edge of the skin. Note that the sutures in the upper skin edge were taken transversely while those on the edge of the areola were horizontal. This modification of the technique was made to accommodate for the length difference between the 2 edges. See Figure 9.8.

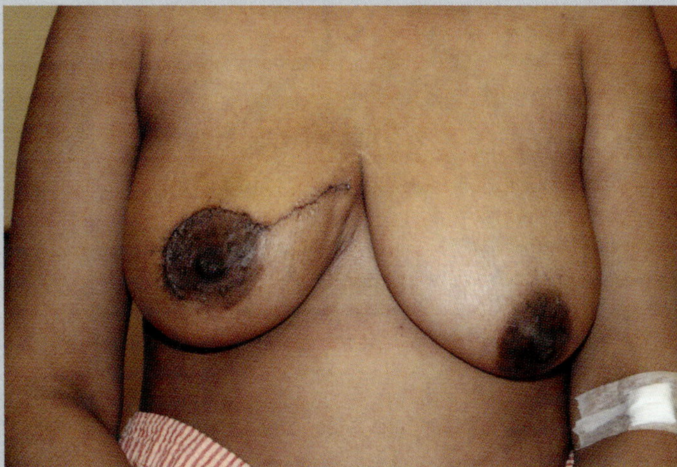

Image 2.6. The patient 2 weeks postoperatively. Notice that the technique used to approximate the edge of the dome has resulted in a very satisfactory cosmetic result in spite of the difference in lengths.

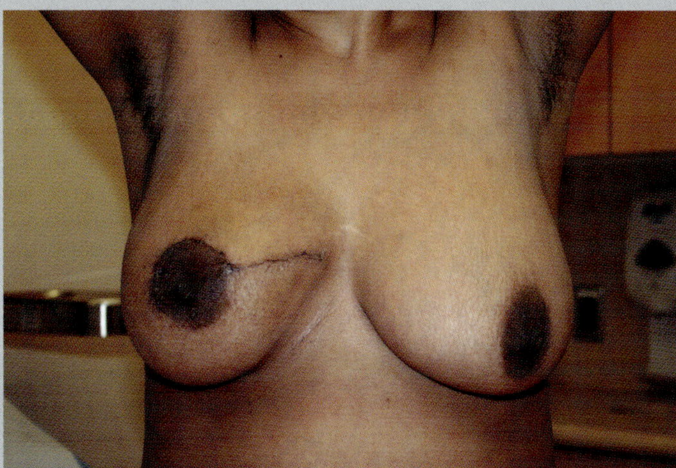

Image 2.7. The patient 2 weeks postoperatively. The contralateral procedure was delayed awaiting completion of radiation therapy.

The resection of the primary, as well as the closure of the defect, follows the same principles described in Chapter 6. Skin closure of the dome does not follow the classical principles as the outer part of the ellipse or the dome is longer than the inner part. We close these wounds by using transverse dermal sutures on the upper flaps and a vertical suture on the lower flap (Figure 9.8) (Case 2, Image 2.5). The final postoperative result

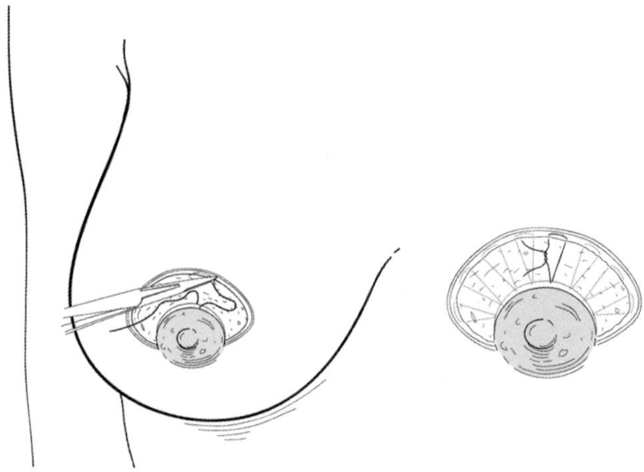

Figure 9.8. Suturing of the dome skin. Multiple interrupted sutures are applied to distribute the discrepancy in size. The suture is taken transversely deep in the dermis of the longer segment of the dome and vertically at the aerolar edge (the shorter segment). A continuous subcuticular closure is then applied in the superficial dermis. See Case No. 2, Images 2.5 and 2.6 for a clinical demonstration.

is cosmetically acceptable (Case 2, Images 2.6 and 2.7). With the batwing technique, the lengths of the upper and lower flaps are equal, and a regular skin closure would be applied.

## 9.3 Benelli Mastopexy

This eponymous technique was first described and popularized by Dr. Louis Benelli.[6] The procedure was designed to minimize scarring in breast surgery. In a Benelli mastopexy, the skin incision starts with a circumareolar design surrounded by a tear drop-shaped incision. The tear drop-shaped incision is drawn using the following criteria (Figure 9.9):

1. The new position of the apex of the areola should be the apex of the tear drop (point A).
2. The distance of the lower edge of the areola from the inframammary line is the bottom of the tear drop (point B).
3. The width of the tear drop depends on the extent of skin excess to be excised. (Line CD).

More recently, some oncoplastic surgeons have adopted this procedure with some modifications using a circumferential periareolar incision with a surrounding ellipse [Figure 9.10(a)] or a second surrounding circle [Figure 9.10(b)], better known as "donut mastopexy."

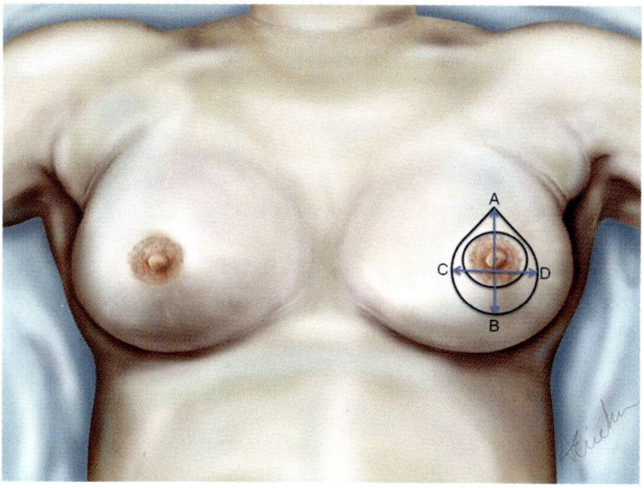


Figure 9.9. Benelli mastopexy as originally described by Louis Benelli.[6]

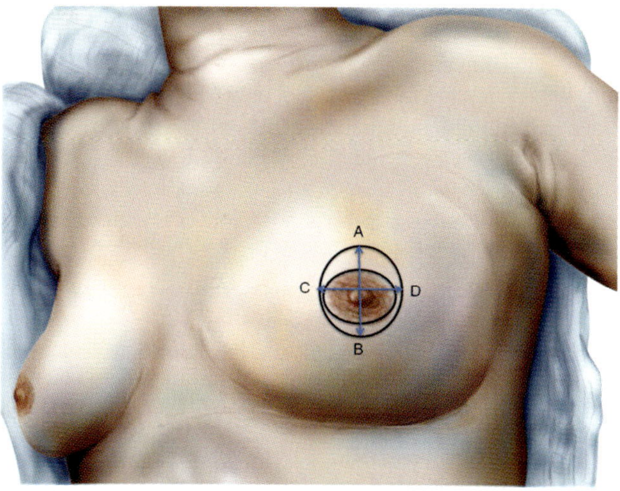


(a)

Figure 9.10. Modified Benelli mastopexy. (a) The outer incision line is elliptical.

The first circle is around the edge of the areola or centered around the nipple; its diameter depends on the desired final size of the new areola. The outer ellipse or circle is directly related to the extent of skin resection needed to tighten the skin envelope of the breast and the desired elevation of the nipple areola complex using the same principles for the Benelli tear drop points A,B,C, and D in Figure 9.9.

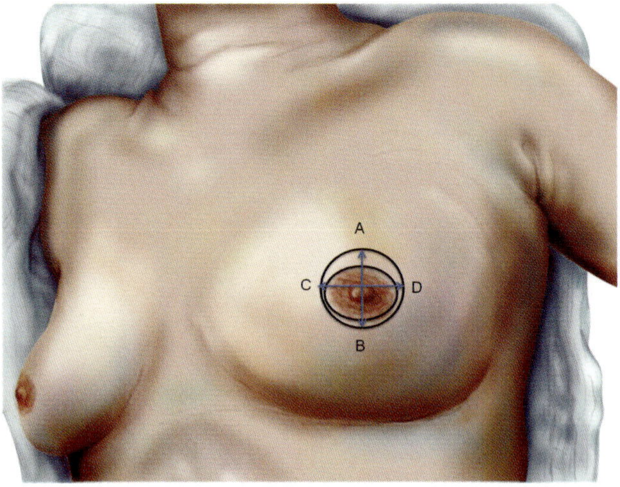


(b)

Figure 9.10. (b) The outer incision line is a second circle, better known as "donut mastopexy."

The skin between the larger circle or ellipse and the outer edge of the inner circle is de-epithelialized rather than excised, therefore maintaining the blood and nerve supply of the nipple areola complex (Case 2, Image 2.4). The skin incision through the dermis and subcutaneous tissue is made at the edge of the outer circle. The skin is elevated, exposing the underlying breast tissue. This procedure gives access to any quadrant. The lumpectomy is then performed. The breast tissue is approximated radially with 2-0 or 3-0 Vicryl as described in Chapter 7. The skin edge at the outer circle is pulled toward the edge of the areola and approximated to each other in 2 layers. As described in the dome mastopexy closure, the length of the outer edge is longer than the inner edge; therefore we recommend using the same technique of approximation previously described: transverse suture on the outer edge and vertical suture on the inner edge (Figure 9.8). Originally, Benelli described his mastopexy as using a continuous non-absorbable sub-cuticular suture to approximate the 2 edges of skin. More recently, many surgeons have abandoned this this type of approximation and resort to 2 layers of closure, an interrupted deep dermal layer as described in Figure 9.8, followed by a continuous mono-filament sub-cuticular layer.

The donut mastopexy can be combined with a full-thickness radial resection in the lower quadrants as shown in Figure 9.11. Such a combination is usually the basis of the J-mastopexy. Such combinations of donut mastopexy and radial resection may be applied to any quadrant in

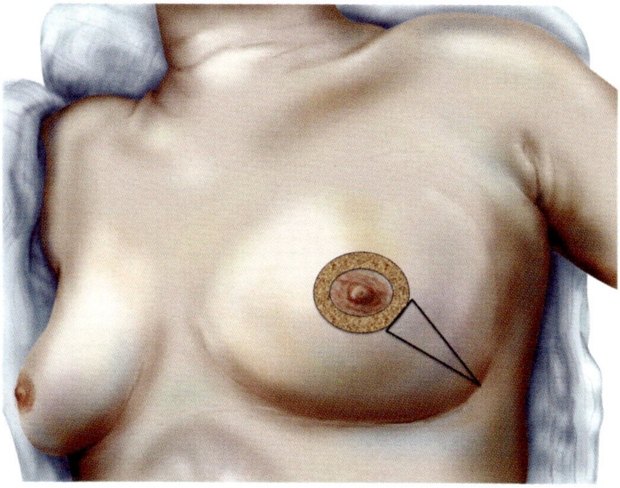

Figure 9.11. Combining donut mastopexy with resection of lesions in the lower outer quadrant in the form of a J-mastopexy.

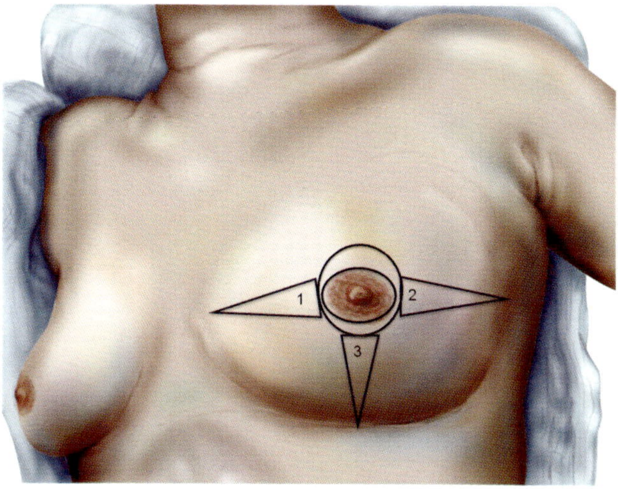


Figure 9.12. Benelli mastopexy with radial extensions: Any of these extensions (1, 2, or 3) could be used with a Benelli procedure.

the breast (Figure 9.12). As we have previously stated in Chapter 4, we avoid radial incisions between 11 o′clock and 2 o′clock axes on the right side, and the 9 o′clock and 1 o′clock axes on the left (Figure 4.3), as they may result in unsightly scars.

For further reading on the subject of more-complex reduction and mastopexy, please refer to Chapter 8: Oncoplastic Breast Reduction.

We strongly recommend that breast/general surgeons who are novices in these complex procedures collaborate with their plastic surgery colleagues.

## References

1. Silverstein MJ. (2003) An argument against routine use of radiotherapy for ductal carcinoma *in situ*. *Oncology (Williston Park)*. 17(11):1511–1533.
2. Berry MG, Fitoussi AD, Cutnier A, Couturaud B, Salmon RJ. (2010) Oncoplastic breast surgery: A review and systematic approach. *J Plast Reconst Aesthet Surg* 63:1233–1243.
3. Fitoussi A, Berry MG, Couturaud B, Salmon RJ. (2009) Oncoplastic breast surgery. *Oncoplastic and Reconstructive Surgery for Breast Cancer. The Institut Curie Experience.* Springer-Verlag, Berlin, Heidelberg.
4. Silverstein MJ. (2009) Oncoplastic breast conservation surgery. In: Nahabedian MY (ed.), *Oncoplastic Surgery of the Breast*, Elsevier, China, pp. 47–70.
5. Fitoussi A, Berry MG, Couturaud B, Salmon RJ. (2009) Oncoplastic breast surgery. P. 29 Figure (a-b). In: *Oncoplastic and Reconstructive Surgery for Breast Cancer. The Institut Curie Experience*, Springer-Verlag, Berlin, Heidelberg.
6. Benelli L. (1990) A new periareolar mammaplasty: The "round block" technique. *Aesthet Plast Surg* 14:93–100.

# Chapter 10

# SKIN-SPARING MASTECTOMY

Walter Paul Weber and Mahmoud El-Tamer

*Breast Service, Department of Surgery,*
*Memorial Sloan-Kettering Cancer Center,*
*New York, NY 10065, USA*

## 10.1 Introduction

The original technique of skin-sparing mastectomy (SSM) for removal of malignant tumors was first described by Toth and Lappert in 1991.[1] While the exact definition of SSM continues to be the subject of discussion, the procedure generally involves the removal of the entire gland, together with the nipple areola complex (NAC) and any biopsy scars, while preserving most if not all of the overlying skin.[2] The preservation of the skin envelope and the inframammary fold (IMF) allows for maintaining the shape of the breast for immediate reconstruction and still provides access to the axilla for possible lymph node dissection. Hence, SSM can be performed as a total mastectomy or as a modified radical mastectomy.

The success of the SSM procedure depends largely on the meticulous preservation of the blood supply to the skin flaps. The anatomy of the arterial system irrigating the skin overlying the breast was described as early as 1939 in Salmon's landmark anatomic studies on the main arteries of the female breast in deceased women between 20 and 45 years of age.[3] The internal thoracic artery is the main artery of supply via perforators through the second, third, and fourth intercostal spaces. A principal vessel passes through the second or third space, giving off many branches to the superficial fascia and skin. An equally significant contribution comes from branches of the lateral thoracic artery or from the superficial thoracic artery directly off the axillary artery. These vessels enter the breast in the upper outer quadrant and give branches to the skin. Superiorly, there may be an additional contribution from the cutaneous branches of the thoracoacromial axis (for details, see Chapter 1).

## 10.2 Incision

The most common approaches are the elliptical incision (Figure 10.1), and the circumareolar incision (Figure 10.2) with medial and/or lateral extensions when the areolar diameter is small (Figure 10.3).[4–6] Figure 10.4 shows a clinical example of elliptical, circumareolar and circumareolar incisions with lateral and medial extensions. In large- or ptotic-breasted women, a Wise-pattern incision may be an option (Figure 10.5). Alternatively, a reduction mammoplasty or mastopexy incision can be used (Figure 10.6). Excess skin can be excised around the areola, and an extension may be added in the form of a J-mastopexy. Modifications include lateral extensions — commonly referred to as "tennis racquet" or "fish-tail" (Figures 10.7–10.8) incisions — to facilitate access to the axilla. Some surgeons prefer a separate axillary incision.[7,8] We have frequently used a separate axillary incision when performing a circumareolar incision without any extension. The type of incision is ultimately based on the preferences of the breast and the reconstructive surgeons and, as such, should be planned by both in agreement. The incision is determined by multiple factors, including the need for skin resection (skin involvement of retraction), the size and

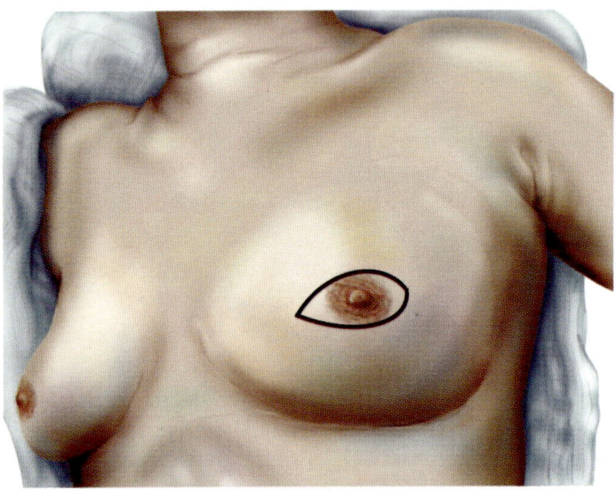

Figure 10.1. Elliptical incision: An ellipse is drawn around the areola. This type of incision is chosen most frequently when using a breast implant for reconstruction.

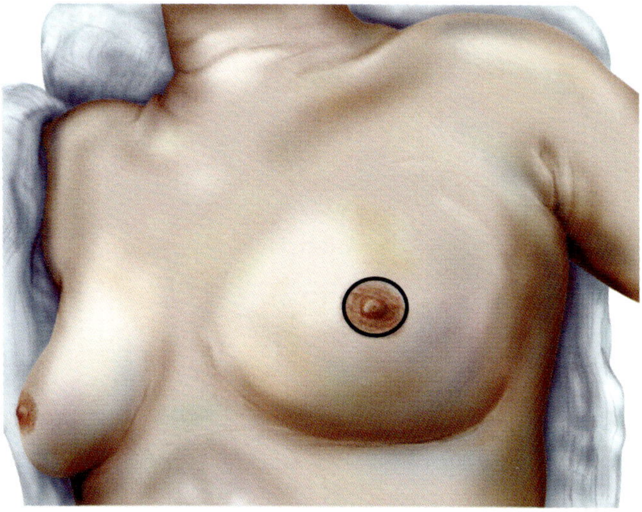

Figure 10.2. The circumareolar incision is ideal for patients who undergo breast reconstruction with tissue transfer. The skin of the myocutaneous flap will be limited to replace the resected areola and will be used to reconstruct the nipple. Such reconstruction achieves an excellent cosmetic result (see Figure 10.8). It is occasionally used with implant reconstruction, and the skin is closed with a purse-string suture.

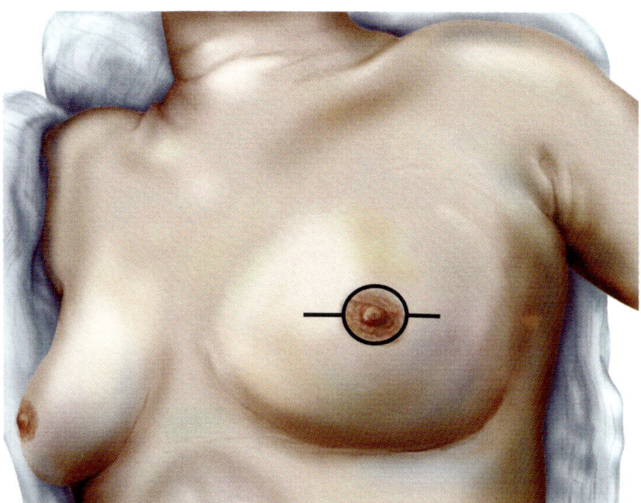

Figure 10.3. The circumareolar incision with lateral/medial extension is also ideal for large-breasted patients who are undergoing breast reconstruction with tissue transfer. It also may facilitate access to axillary node dissection or biopsy (see Figure 10.9).

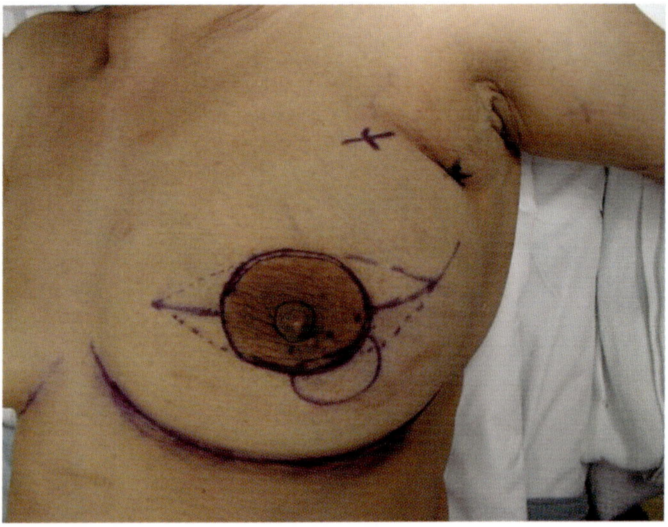

Figure 10.4. The patient on the OR table with drawings of elliptical, circumareolar, and circumareolar incisions with lateral and/or medial extensions.

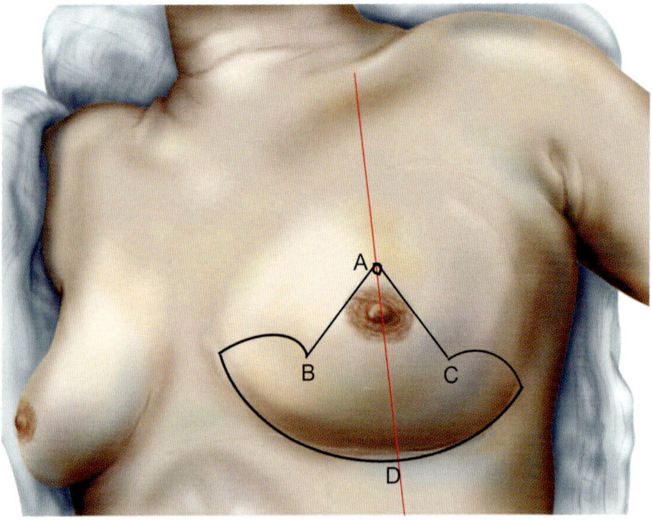


Figure 10.5. The Wise pattern: Applicable to patients with ptotic breasts who will require resection of excess skin. One of the major concerns of such an incision is the limited ability to expand the skin over the inverted T scar. We have frequently used such incisions in patients who have undergone recent breast reductions.

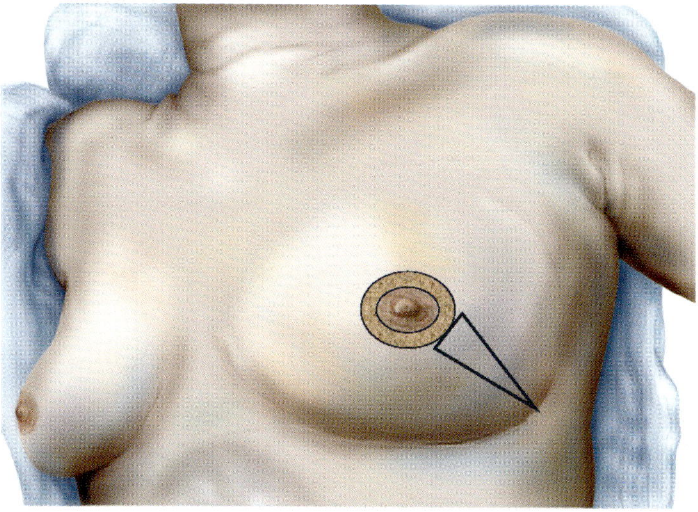

Figure 10.6. This type of incision is favored in patients who have ptotic breasts with excess skin and who are planned for tissue transfer reconstruction. The excess skin of the breast may be taken around the areola with or without a lateral extension in the form of a J-mastopexy.

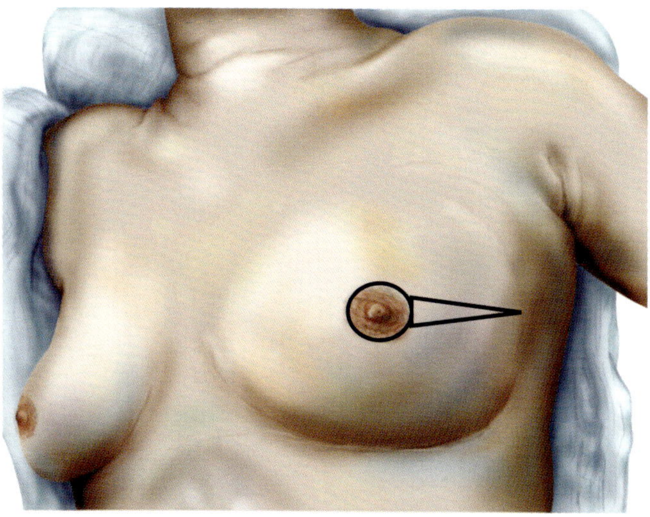

Figure 10.7. "Fish-tail" or "tennis racquet" incisions are very helpful when planning resection of the skin or prior lumpectomy scars. The triangular extension is centered around the area of skin to be excised. The triangular extension may be aligned toward any quadrant of the breast as seen in Figure 10.8.

degree of ptosis of the breast, the diameter of the areola, prior lumpectomy scars, and type of reconstruction (autologous versus implants).

For patients with planned autologous tissue transfer, we prefer the circumareolar incision because it results in minimal scarring with optimal cosmetic results (Figure 10.9). When planning reconstruction with an expander, we have resorted to an elliptical incision because circumareolar incisions are usually converted to elliptical for closure. Regardless of the

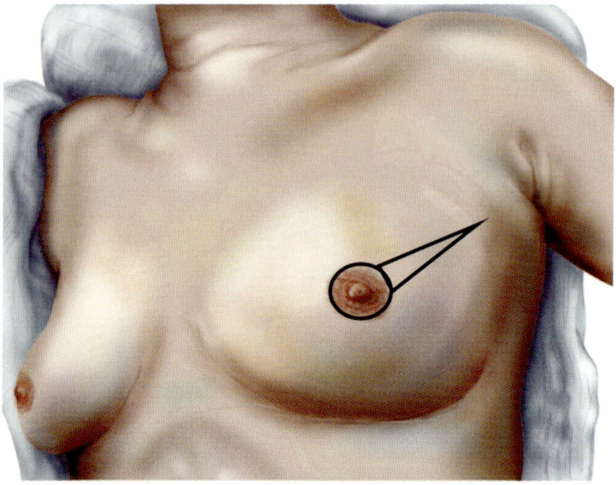

Figure 10.8. "Fish tail" with triangular extension to the upper outer quadrant.

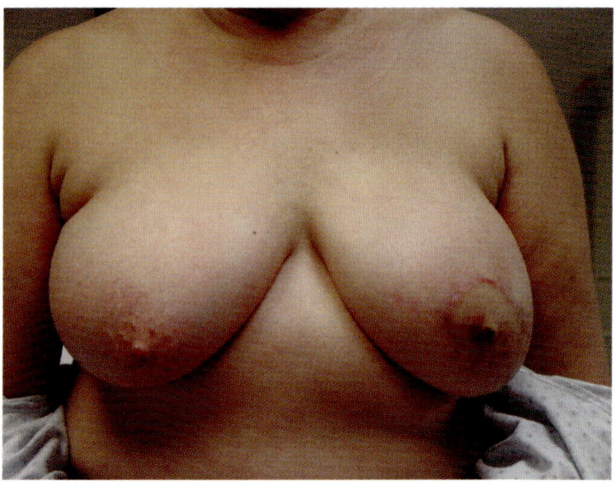

Figure 10.9. This patient underwent a skin-sparing total mastectomy through a circumareolar incision with bilateral extension.

type of incision used, however, the primary goal remains complete oncologic resection. Therefore, additional skin removal may be necessary to achieve clear anterior margins.

## 10.3 Mastectomy

The same mastectomy principles used in a non-SSM apply to SSM. When the circumareolar incision is used, however, the procedure can become challenging in patients with a small NAC and rigid skin; we have frequently resorted to lateral/medial extensions in these cases. Early, in the experience of breast surgeons, we recommend extending the lateral incisions without skin resection to achieve a complete extirpation of the breast. The patient is placed supine with the arm extended on a padded arm board. The arm should be prepped and draped separately to allow free rotation. After the skin incision is completed, the subcutaneous planes are exposed. Hemostasis should be maintained at all times during the procedure. Dissection may be performed with electrocautery or by sharp dissection with scalpel or curved scissors. If sharp dissection is undertaken, the tumescent mastectomy technique significantly reduces bleeding. This procedure refers to the subcutaneous injection of a liquid mixture of salts and small amounts of two drugs: lidocaine to numb the area, and epinephrine to narrow the blood vessels and reduce bleeding. We use a solution which consists of 1,000 ml of Ringers lactate with 20 cc of 1% lidocaine with epinephrine 1:100,000.

Retractors, clamps, or skin hooks are used to elevate the skin edges. We strongly recommend following the superficial fascial plane while elevating the skin flaps (see Chapter 1). Dissection in that plane is bloodless and preserves the integrity of the blood supply to the overlying skin. Adhering to the superficial fascial plane is a crucial factor to the survival of the skin flaps and maximal removal of breast tissue. We avoid adhering to a specific thickness when elevating the skin flaps as there is significant variation between patients. Furthermore, the skin flaps in the same patient gradually increase in thickness while moving away from the NAC. Although some have doubted the presence of a superficial fascial plane and have not been able to identify it as a histologic entity,[9] we feel that in a significant number of patients, the subcutaneous plane is well visualized when raising the flaps. In some patients, however, we have found some difficulty in clearly identifying that "bloodless" plane.

To identify the plane of dissection, the assistant holds upward tension on the skin flaps while the surgeon uses countertraction on the breast parenchyma. Excessive bleeding indicates that the dissection is not in the correct anatomic plane that separates the superficial fascia from the subdermal vascular plexus. Special caution should be exercised to preserve the principal blood vessels of the skin, and a profound knowledge of the vascular anatomy of the skin overlying the breast (as summarized in the introduction of this chapter) is mandatory for the success of the SSM procedure. The skin flaps extend superiorly to the clavicle, medially to the sternal edge, and laterally to the latissimus dorsi. The lower skin flap is then developed to the inframammary crease. There have been reports in the literature describing the importance of maintaining the IMF. We have routinely used the same technique for SSM and conventional mastectomy. The IMF can be recreated by imbricating the skin to the chest wall during the reconstructive procedure.

In non-SSM, we have traditionally started with the upper flap and addressed the lower flap later. In SSM, however, our experience consists of progressively raising the flaps circumferentially. We recommend using deep Richardson retractors or, preferably, lighted 90-degree retractors.

The next step is the removal of the breast. We start superiorly and progress downward along the pectoralis muscle fibers. We have routinely included the pectoralis fascia based on the anatomic observation of breast tissue extending to the fascia through Cooper's ligament. In prophylactic mastectomy, however, we may keep the pectoralis fascia intact and adhere to the retromammary space. Many small arteries perforate the pectoralis muscle and contribute to the circulation of the breast; we recommend careful cauterization of these vessels. Of note, however, are the medial parasternal perforators, particularly those that arise from the second or third intercostal spaces: the internal mammary perforators. These vessels are relatively larger in caliber, and we recommend taking the time to ligate or clip these vessels. The dissection is extended to the lateral aspect of the pectoralis major and serratus muscles, and the breast is removed. We have found that elevating the skin off the axillary breast tail to be quite difficult through a circumareolar incision. We address the axillary tail after having raised the superior, medial, and inferior flaps, and after separating the breast off of the muscle. The breast is exteriorized through the nipple areola defect and used for traction. This technical maneuver facilitates raising the skin flaps of the axillary tail and dissecting the axilla. We routinely apply a suture in the axillary tail for specimen orientation prior to submission for pathologic evaluation.

## 10.4 Axillary Staging

Extensions are usually not necessary for adequate access to the sentinel lymph nodes. All blue and/or "hot" lymph nodes are removed, along with any suspicious, palpable nodes. For complete axillary lymph node dissection, the breast envelope is reflected laterally to gain access to the axilla. If access is difficult, "tennis racquet", "fish-tail", or separate axillary incisions allow easier exposure. Typically, the reduction incision and modified ellipse allow good access to the axilla without extensions. Axillary lymph node dissection clears levels I and II. Complete axillary clearance that includes levels I, II, and III is only indicated when the surgeon palpates suspicious nodes in the apex of the axilla. When relying on blue dye to identify the sentinel node, we strongly recommend a separate axillary incision.

## 10.5 Reconstruction

Reconstruction can be performed with an implant or with a tissue transfer, preferably with autologous tissue from the abdominal wall (TRAM flap/DIEP flap) or back (latissimus flap). Typically, with an implant reconstruction, a tissue expander is placed at the time of the SSM under the pectoralis muscle. The tissue expander is injected with saline over few weeks to stretch the subpectoral pocket. The permanent implant is placed during a second procedure. In patients who are having an autologous reconstruction, we have exerted every effort to limit our incision to around the areola. The plastic surgeon then limits the skin paddle of the flap to the NAC defect

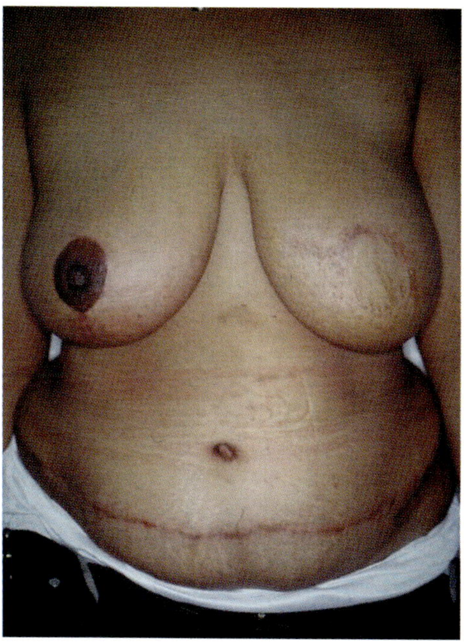

Figure 10.10. Circumareolar incision. The abdominal skin paddle is limited to the site of the NAC.

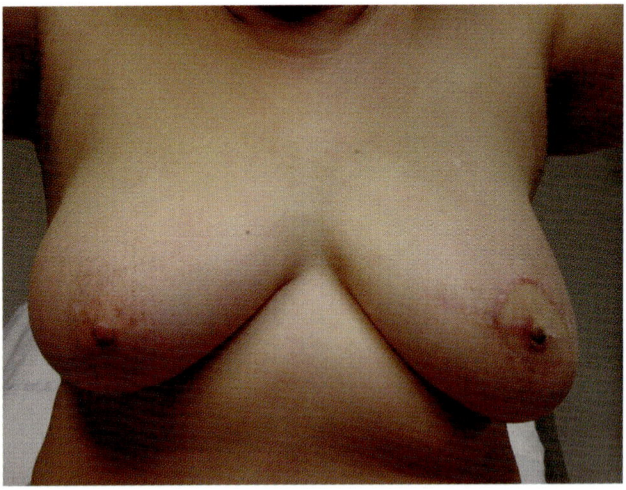

Figure 10.11. Flap skin paddle used to reconstruct the nipple and tattooed as an areola.

(Figure 10.10). The myocutaneous flap skin paddle can later be used to reconstruct the nipple and tattooed as an areola. In our experience this technique has led to excellent cosmetic results (Figure 10.11).

## 10.6 Safety

Safety of the SSM technique can be defined in 3 ways. The first is the risk of short-term complications which may delay adjuvant therapy. The second is the risk of incompleteness of mastectomy due to limited exposure compared with the non-SSM technique, hence leaving residual breast tissue behind that may be prone for future malignant transformation, particularly in mutation carriers and high-risk patients. The third is the risk of incompleteness of tumor removal in the skin envelope, resulting in positive margins. All of these factors could, in theory, jeopardize the oncologic outcome in terms of local recurrence.

## 10.7 Postoperative Complications

Aside from reconstructive procedure complications, the principal postoperative concern is skin-flap ischemia. This occurs in 5% to 15% of patients and ranges from simple epidermolysis to full-thickness skin flap necrosis.[10–12] The resulting exposure of muscle or implant may cause skin retractions, infection, or even loss of the implant. The latter has been reported in up to 18% of patients.[4,11–13] Therefore every effort should be made to preserve the main blood supply to the skin of the female breast. Other complications include hematoma and seroma, which occur in the initial postoperative period.[14]

A recent study assessed potential risk factors for postoperative complications and found that the Wise-pattern and the "tennis racquet" incision had significantly higher rates of wound dehiscence when compared with the circumareolar incision ($p = 0.025$ and $p = 0.098$, respectively).[15] There was no significant difference between diathermy or blade dissection techniques, and no higher risk associated with the use of the tumescent mastectomy technique. However, recent studies have shown higher wound complication with the tumescent technique in patients undergoing mastectomy and immediate reconstruction.[16]

## 10.8 Completeness of Mastectomy

The goal in all mastectomies is to create skin flaps that are thin enough to remove all breast tissue and thick enough to provide sufficient blood supply. The amount of breast tissue left behind, however, is similar in both SSM and non-SSM techniques.[9] In patients undergoing SSM, residual glandular tissue is found in more than one-half of the patients in the IMF, but this accounts for only 0.02% of total breast tissue.[17] Hence there is no evidence in the literature suggesting that SSM is less complete than non-SSM.

## 10.9 Completeness of Tumor Removal and Local Recurrence Rates

The main oncologic concern in SSM relates to the possibility of leaving residual tumor within the skin envelope, which may manifest later as local recurrence. Ho *et al.*[18] performed a histological analysis on the skin and 10 mm of the subcutaneous tissue of 30 total mastectomy specimens by the step-serial–sectioning technique. They found that the incidence of skin-flap involvement outside the NAC was 23% (7 of 30). The significant parameters related to skin-flap involvement were skin tethering (75% versus 15%, $p < 0.05$), pathologic tumor size ($p < 0.03$), and perineural infiltration (63% versus 9%, $p < 0.01$). The authors concluded that it would be oncologically safe to perform SSM in T1 and T2 tumors, and preserve the skin overlying the tumor, if there is no skin tethering.

Even though the previously cited study provided indirect evidence of the appropriateness of SSM, the oncologic safety of SSM is ultimately

Table 10.1. Local recurrence rates after skin-sparing mastectomy versus non-skin–sparing mastectomy.

| Study | Median follow-up (months) | N (SSM) | LR in SSM (%) | N (non-SSM) | LR in non-SSM (%) |
|---|---|---|---|---|---|
| Carlson *et al.*[6] | 42 | 327 | 4.8 | 188 | 9.5 |
| Kroll *et al.*[25] | 72 | 104 | 6.7 | 27 | 7.4 |
| Slavin *et al.*[4] | 45 | 51 | 2.0 | 188 | 9.5 |
| Simmons *et al.*[5] | 60 | 77 | 3.9 | 154 | 3.3 |
| Rivadeneira *et al.*[29] | 49 | 71 | 5.6 | 127 | 3.9 |
| Greenway *et al.*[27] | 49 | 225 | 3.8 | 1022 | 3.9 |
| Howard *et al.*[28] | 59 | 34 | 0 | 395 | 3.8 |
| Gerber *et al.*[35] | 101 | 48 | 10.4 | 130 | 11.5 |

determined by the long-term rates of local recurrence. There are no randomized clinical trials evaluating the safety of SSM to date. In addition, many of the observational studies on SSM reported a mean follow-up of 8–24 months, which seems to be too short for evaluation of oncologic safety.[14,19–25] The vast majority of local recurrence following a total mastectomy occurs within 24 months, however. Multiple observational studies with a sufficient follow-up of longer than 24 months demonstrated low local recurrence rates in patients undergoing SSM for breast cancer.[4–6,26–35] They ranged from 0% to 10.4%, and were similar for the SSM and the non-SSM groups (Table 10.1). Since the majority of these studies included T1-2 and stage 0-II disease, multicentric cancer, ductal carcinoma *in situ*, and risk-reduction surgery, it can be concluded that SSM is safe in these patients. Increasing clinical experience, however, suggests that SSM can be reliably performed in larger tumors as long as there is sufficient distance between the tumor and the skin in the absence of skin changes. This includes large tumors which are downstaged by neoadjuvant CTX. Hence, the only absolute contraindications for SSM in today's surgical practice are inflammatory breast cancer and direct tumor involvement of the skin.

## 10.10 Cosmesis

SSM preserves the breast envelope and facilitates immediate breast reconstruction.[15] Gerber *et al.* have shown that the aesthetic results are better compared with secondary breast reconstruction, and that the improved aesthetic result translates to greater patient and surgeon satisfaction after SSM compared to modified radical mastectomy.[36,37]

Over time, the reconstructed tissue regains the shape of the original breast envelope, allowing symmetry and ptosis to be achieved.[38] SSM prevents transverse scars associated with conventional non-SSM. (Figures 10.10–10.11). In patients who undergo circumareolar incision and tissue reconstruction, the cutaneous part of the flap is only visible as an island for the NAC, thereby preventing contrast between the pale abdominal skin and the breast envelope.[8,39] This provides an ideal color and texture to the breast skin.[14] The best cosmetic outcomes are found in women who have not had prior RT and those who are unlikely to need adjuvant RT, even though RT does not represent a contraindication for SSM and immediate breast reconstruction.[33]

## References


1. Toth BA, Lappert P. (1991) Modified skin incisions for mastectomy: The need for plastic surgical input in preoperative planning. *Plast Reconstr Surg* 87(6):1048–1053.
2. Bleicher RJ, Hansen NM, Giuliano AE. (2003) Skin-sparing mastectomy specialty bias and worldwide lack of consensus. *Cancer* 98(11):2316–2321.
3. Salmon M. Les artères de la glande mammaire. (1939) *Ann Anat Pathol* 16:477–500.
4. Slavin SA, Schnitt SJ, Duda RB, *et al.* (1998) Skin-sparing mastectomy and immediate reconstruction: Oncologic risks and aesthetic results in patients with early-stage breast cancer. *Plast Reconstr Surg* 102(1):49–62.
5. Simmons RM, Fish SK, Gayle L, *et al.* (1999) Local and distant recurrence rates in skin-sparing mastectomies compared with non-skin-sparing mastectomies. *Ann Surg Oncol* 6(7):676–681.
6. Carlson GW, Bostwick J, 3rd, Styblo TM, *et al.* (1997) Skin-sparing mastectomy. Oncologic and reconstructive considerations. *Ann Surg* 225(5):570–575; discussion 575–578.
7. Toth BA, Forley BG, Calabria R. (1999) Retrospective study of the skin-sparing mastectomy in breast reconstruction. *Plast Reconstr Surg* 104(1):77–84.
8. Hidalgo DA. (1998) Aesthetic refinement in breast reconstruction: Complete skin-sparing mastectomy with autogenous tissue transfer. *Plast Reconstr Surg* 102(1):63–70; discussion 71–72.
9. Barton FE, Jr., English JM, Kingsley WB, *et al.* (1991) Glandular excision in total glandular mastectomy and modified radical mastectomy: A comparison. *Plast Reconstr Surg* 88(3):389–392; discussion 393–394.
10. Sufi PA, Gittos M, Collier DS. (2000) Envelope mastectomy with immediate reconstruction (EMIR). *Eur J Surg Oncol* 26(4):367–370.
11. Carlson GW, Losken A, Moore B, *et al.* (2001) Results of immediate breast reconstruction after skin-sparing mastectomy. *Ann Plast Surg* 46(3):222–228.

12. Contant CM, van Geel AN, van der Holt B, *et al.* (2000) Morbidity of immediate breast reconstruction (IBR) after mastectomy by a subpectorally placed silicone prosthesis: The adverse effect of radiotherapy. *Eur J Surg Oncol* 26(4):344–350.
13. Clough KB, Bourgeois D, Falcou MC, *et al.* (1996) Immediate breast reconstruction by prosthesis: A safe technique for extensive intraductal and microinvasive carcinomas. *Ann Surg Oncol* 3(2):212–218.
14. Munhoz AM, Aldrighi C, Montag E, *et al.* (2007) Periareolar skin-sparing mastectomy and latissimus dorsi flap with biodimensional expander implant reconstruction: Surgical planning, outcome, and complications. *Plast Reconstr Surg* 119(6):1637–1649; discussion 1650–1652.
15. Davies AL, Roblin P, Ross D, Farhadi J. (2010) Factors affecting post-operative complications following skin sparing mastectomy with immediate breast reconstruction. *The Breast*; Epub ahead of print.
16. Seth AK, Hirsch EM, Fine NA, Dumanian GA, Mustoe TA, Galiano RD, Hansen NM, Kim JY. (2011) Additive risk of tumescent technique in patients undergoing mastectomy with immediate reconstruction. *Ann Surg Oncol* 18(11):3041–3046.
17. Carlson GW, Grossl N, Lewis MM, *et al.* (1996) Preservation of the inframammary fold: What are we leaving behind? *Plast Reconstr Surg* 98(3): 447–450.
18. Ho CM, Mak CK, Lau Y, *et al.* (2003) Skin involvement in invasive breast carcinoma: Safety of skin-sparing mastectomy. *Ann Surg Oncol* 10(2): 102–107.
19. Margulies AG, Hochberg J, Kepple J, *et al.* (2005) Total skin-sparing mastectomy without preservation of the nipple-areola complex. *Am J Surg* 190(6):907–912.
20. Petit JY, Veronesi U, Orecchia R, *et al.* (2006) Nipple-sparing mastectomy in association with intra operative radiotherapy (ELIOT): A new type of mastectomy for breast cancer treatment. *Breast Cancer Res Treat* 96(1): 47–51.
21. Salhab M, Al Sarakbi W, Joseph A, *et al.* (2006) Skin-sparing mastectomy and immediate breast reconstruction: Patient satisfaction and clinical outcome. *Int J Clin Oncol* 11(1):51–54.
22. Peyser PM, Abel JA, Straker VF, *et al.* (2000) Ultra-conservative skin-sparing 'keyhole' mastectomy and immediate breast and areola reconstruction. *Ann R Coll Surg Engl* 82(4):227–235.
23. Rashid M, Ilahi I, ur Rehman Sarwar S, *et al.* (2005) Skin sparing mastectomy and immediate breast reconstruction. *J Coll Phys Surg Pak* 15(8): 467–471.
24. Psaila A, Pozzi M, Barone Adesi L, *et al.* (2006) Nipple sparing mastectomy with immediate breast reconstruction: A short term analysis of our experience. *J Exp Clin Cancer Res* 25(3):309–312.
25. Wijayanayagam A, Kumar AS, Foster RD, *et al.* (2008) Optimizing the total skin-sparing mastectomy. *Arch Surg* 143(1):38–45; discussion 45.

26. Kroll SS, Schusterman MA, Tadjalli HE, *et al.* (1997) Risk of recurrence after treatment of early breast cancer with skin-sparing mastectomy. *Ann Surg Oncol* 4(3):193–197.
27. Greenway RM, Schlossberg L, Dooley WC. (2005) Fifteen-year series of skin-sparing mastectomy for stage 0 to 2 breast cancer. *Am J Surg* 190(6):918–922.
28. Howard MA, Polo K, Pusic AL, *et al.* (2006) Breast cancer local recurrence after mastectomy and TRAM flap reconstruction: Incidence and treatment options. *Plast Reconstr Surg* 117(5):1381–1386.
29. Rivadeneira DE, Simmons RM, Fish SK, *et al.* (2000) Skin-sparing mastectomy with immediate breast reconstruction: A critical analysis of local recurrence. *Cancer J* 6(5):331–335.
30. Medina-Franco H, Vasconez LO, Fix RJ, *et al.* (2002) Factors associated with local recurrence after skin-sparing mastectomy and immediate breast reconstruction for invasive breast cancer. *Ann Surg* 235(6):814–819.
31. Fersis N, Hoenig A, Relakis K, *et al.* (2004) Skin-sparing mastectomy and immediate breast reconstruction: Incidence of recurrence in patients with invasive breast cancer. *Breast* 13(6):488–493.
32. Downes KJ, Glatt BS, Kanchwala SK, *et al.* (2005) Skin-sparing mastectomy and immediate reconstruction is an acceptable treatment option for patients with high-risk breast carcinoma. *Cancer* 103(5):906–913.
33. Patani N, Devalia H, Anderson A, *et al.* (2008) Oncological safety and patient satisfaction with skin-sparing mastectomy and immediate breast reconstruction. *Surg Oncol* 17(2):97–105.
34. Omranipour R, Bobin JY, Esouyeh M. (2008) Skin Sparing Mastectomy and Immediate Breast Reconstruction (SSMIR) for early breast cancer: Eight years single institution experience. *World J Surg Oncol* 6:43.
35. Gerber B, Krause A, Dieterich M, *et al.* (2009) The oncological safety of skin sparing mastectomy with conservation of the nipple-areola complex and autologous reconstruction: An extended follow-up study. *Ann Surg* 249(3):461–468.
36. Gerber B, Krause A, Kuchenmeister I, *et al.* (2000) Skin sparing mastectomy with autologous immediate reconstruction: Oncological risks and aesthetic results. *Zentralbl Gynakol* 122(9):476–482.
37. Gerber B, Krause A, Reimer T, *et al.* (2003) Skin-sparing mastectomy with conservation of the nipple-areola complex and autologous reconstruction is an oncologically safe procedure. *Ann Surg* 238(1):120–127.
38. Sotheran WJ, Rainsbury RM. (2004) Skin-sparing mastectomy in the UK — A review of current practice. *Ann R Coll Surg Engl* 86(2):82–86.
39. Bensimon RH, Bergmeyer JM. (1995) Improved aesthetics in breast reconstruction: Modified mastectomy incision and immediate autologous tissue reconstruction. *Ann Plast Surg* 34(3):229–233; discussion 233–235.

# Chapter 11

# NIPPLE-SPARING MASTECTOMY

Sunny Mitchell* and Sheldon Marc Feldman†

**Women's Breast Center, Department of Surgery, Tully Health Center, 32 Strawberry Hill Court, Stamford, CT 06902, USA*

*†Division of Breast Surgical Oncology, Columbia University Medical Center, New York City, NY, 10032, USA*

## 11.1 Introduction

Nipple-sparing mastectomy (NSM) entails removing all breast tissue, including all breast tissue immediately under the nipple areola complex (NAC), while sparing the skin envelope, including the NAC. This type of mastectomy, combined with immediate reconstruction, leads to a postoperative reconstructed breast, appearing nearly identical to a preoperative breast (unless a mastopexy is added to decrease ptosis). Benefits include nipple and areola preservation, and improved overall cosmesis. This is in direct contrast to the more traditional mastectomy types — modified radical mastectomy (MRM), total mastectomy (TM), or skin-sparing mastectomy (SSM) — all of which entail removing the NAC with varying amounts of skin immediately surrounding the NAC. A subcutaneous mastectomy has been described as a mastectomy which entails sparing the NAC as well as a variable amount of breast tissue. Ideally, NSM removes all detectable breast tissue.

Historically, concerns regarding sparing the NAC included oncologic safety, technical difficulty, aesthetics (final nipple position), and viability of the nipple. There has been a growing acceptance of the procedural utility of NSM. The guidelines utilized in deciding which patients are appropriate candidates for NSM are based on metrics used to preoperatively predict a lack of NAC involvement and the anticipation of an acceptable cosmetic result.

## 11.2 Rationale

The rationale for this type of mastectomy is straightforward. The ability to perform a mastectomy in a woman while leaving the NAC in place allows surgeons to accomplish 2 goals: to achieve optimal oncologic surgical treatment and to markedly improve aesthetic outcome. The basis of routinely removing the NAC is increasingly being brought into question as a necessary aspect of the mastectomy.

The psychological benefit of being able to undergo NSM with immediate reconstruction aids in facilitating the healing/recovery process as incidence rates of depression and anxiety can be markedly elevated at the time of a breast cancer diagnosis. Sparing the NAC potentially leads to greater patient satisfaction, body image, and psychological adjustment.[1,2] Women report feeling a "psychological calmness and wholeness" as well as a more natural appearance in relation to opting for NSM.[3] Petit *et al.* reported a total of 91% of patients feeling "less mutilated" by choosing NSM.[4] Many women who undergo SSMs never undergo subsequent nipple areolar creation. They therefore never achieve a near-normal breast appearance.

## 11.3 Why Not Perform NSM?

The standard mastectomy entailed removing the NAC, and routine NAC excision was based on a presumption of possible NAC involvement, concern for NAC viability, and risk of recurrence. An improved understanding of nipple anatomy and disease extent has led to the understanding that this is often unnecessary. Although the NAC can be reconstructed after a non-NSM, many women do not opt to undergo this procedure. Maintaining the native NAC results in a superior cosmetic result compared with a reconstructed NAC. Issues that arise include tattoo fading and variability in the long-term appearance of the reconstructed nipple. Preserving the main landmark of the breast, the NAC, allows breast cancer patients to feel "more intact" and experience better aesthetic outcomes. In the setting of mastectomy, the ability to provide NSM with immediate reconstruction enables the surgical team to provide a postoperative mastectomy breast nearly identical to its preoperative appearance. Here we discuss the role of NSM with a focus on basic science, patient selection, preoperative evaluation, intraoperative technique, and outcomes.

## 11.4 Most Frequently Cited Landmark Study

When discussing the role of NSM, many people point to the series of subcutaneous mastectomies performed at the Mayo Clinic from 1960 to 1993.[5]

In this study, subcutaneous mastectomies were defined as removing ≥90% of breast tissue and leaving residual tissue beneath the NAC. This was a cohort of 639 prophylactic mastectomies performed on moderate- and high-risk (Gail model) patients. After a 14-year follow-up, they reported an 89.5% risk reduction ($p < 0.001$) in the moderate-risk group and a 90% risk reduction in the high-risk group. They also noted no difference in breast cancer incidence between TM and subcutaneous mastectomy. To reiterate, NSM attempts to remove all breast tissue, whereas a subcutaneous mastectomy may not.

## 11.5 Basic Science

### 11.5.1 *Breast Ductal Anatomy*

The median number of ducts is 23. There is no correlation between duct number and age, breast volume, or nipple diameter. A number of ducts commonly share fewer common openings to the nipple surface.[6] Neither duct position nor duct diameter are predictive of whether a system passes deep within the breast or terminates near the nipple.[6] Mean nipple diameter is 11.1 mm. Mean duct bundle diameter is 5.2 mm.[6]

Although the goal is to remove all tissue under the nipple, it is interesting to note that Rusby *et al.*[6] reported that leaving a 2 mm peripheral rim of tissue below the nipple resulted in complete duct excision 96% of the time and 50% retension of microvasculature. The strongest oncologic argument against sparing the NAC has traditionally been the possibility of cancer either originating or recurring within the nipple. Studies have demonstrated NAC involvement in specimens from non-NSMs 10%–25% of the time.[7–10]

### 11.5.2 *The Terminal Ductal Lobular Unit*

Perhaps the most salient support stems from the status of terminal ductal lobular units (TDLUs). As most breast cancers originate in the TDLU, it is important to know if there are TDLUs in the nipple. A study by Stolier *et al.* found that out of 32 mastectomy specimens from 22 patients [prophylactic, 22; invasive ductal carcinoma (IDC), 4; invasive lobular carcinoma (ILC), 1; ductal carcinoma *in situ* (DCIS), 5], only 3 of the 32 specimens had TDLUs at the base of the nipple (1, 2, and 3 TDLUs, respectively). No TDLUs were found at the tip.[7]

## 11.6 Proposed Metrics

Ideally, we would be able to refer to a prospective randomized study comparing NSM and non-NSM. This is unlikely to be performed, however,

Table 11.1. Patient selection metrics.

| | |
|---|---|
| Banerjee[7] | Stages (I,II,II), peripheral tumors <5 cm, irrespective of nodal status or skin involvement |
| Rusby[10] | Multivariable logistic regression model |
| Loewen[13] | Mammographic distance of tumor to NAC <4.96 cm correlates w/NAC involvement. |
| Voltura[25] | Careful pathologic assessment of subareolar breast tissue at surgery. |
| Crowe[26] | Tumor size <3.5 cm; peripheral; no NCT. |
| Crowe[27] | Tumor size <3.5 cm; peripheral; no NCT. |
| Yueh[3] | Tumors <2 cm diameter and >2.5 cm from NAC; no skin or nipple involvement. |
| Petit[19] | Tumor >1 cm from NAC; absence of retroareolar calcs; no bloody nipple discharge, multifocality ok. |
| Petit[20] | Multifocality ok. |
| Wijayanayagam[24] | MRI >2 cm from nipple; small peripheral tumors; no skin involvement. |
| Sacchini[28] | Exclude gross NAC involvement and <1 cm radiograph from areolar margin. |
| Lagios[29] | Tumor >2.5 cm of NAC; tumor size <2 cm. |
| Brachtel[9] | Negative retroareolar margin, HER2 status, size, distance to NAC, lymphovascular invasion, node involvement, histologic grade. |

because the current worldwide experience suggests that many surgeons and patients are increasingly endorsing this approach. We can evaluate the metrics that have been utilized thus far in patient selection (Table 11.1). Proposed factors that may aid in identifying good NSM candidates (those who are the least likely to have NAC involvement) include smaller tumor size, lack of gross involvement of the nipple, distance of tumor from the NAC, peripheral versus central location, radiographic distance from the NAC, and cancer-free core (infra-NAC specimen) tissue.

There are multiple clinical series, reported in the literature, and unpublished international series with results demonstrating acceptably low recurrence risk (Table 11.2). Fukuma *et al.* cite a recurrence rate of <1% within the NAC at 15 years follow-up of over 1,000 patients.[11]

The prospective registry of NSMs sponsored by the American Society of Breast Surgeons Mastery of Breast Surgery Program will provide outcome measures as well as help in delineating ideal metrics.[9] This should prove to be a robust data set.

Formulas[10] and predictive models have been proposed for NAC involvement in NSMs; Rusby *et al.*[10] proposed a multivariable logistic regression model for predicting NAC involvement in NSMs, and Loewen *et al.*[13] proposed a logistic regression equation with NAC involvement as the

Table 11.2. Reported risk of recurrence.

| | Total no. of nipple-sparing mastectomies | Recurrence rate |
|---|---|---|
| Garwood[30] | 170 | |
| Voltura[25] | 51 | 5.90% |
| Sookhan[23] | 18 | 0 |
| Gerber[32] | 60 | 11.70% |
| Crowe[27] | 149 | 4 of 149 |
| Sacchini[28] | 123 | 4 of 123 |
| Regolo[22] | 70 | 0 |
| Ueda[2] | 33 | 5.00% |
| Petit[4] | 773 | 1.50% |
| Petit[20] | 579 | 0.90% per year |
| Petit[19] | 1001 | 1.40% |
| Petit[18] | 300 | 2 of 300 |

*Note*: Petit,[4,18–20] received Intraoperative Radiation with Electrons (ELIOT).

dependent variable, and mammographic distance from the NAC as the independent variable.

## 11.7 Selection

The majority of papers published thus far have proposed (mostly through retrospective reviews and small populations) assessing the following metrics when selecting patients for NSMs: Peripheral versus central tumors; smaller versus larger tumors; presence or lack of skin involvement; nodal status; and indication (prophylaxis, carcinoma, DCIS, and breast cancer [BRCA] status) (Table 11.1). Recurrence rates have been unremarkable (Table 11.2).

Ueda *et al.*[2] found no statistically significant recurrence rate in a comparison of breast-conserving treatment (BCT), TM, and NSM with patients undergoing NSM or BCT, and noted greater overall patient satisfaction in treatment choice. There have been no documented cases of recurrence in the nipple when the tissue immediately underlying the NAC was negative for cancer. Size, shape, and degree of ptosis are important factors to consider when evaluating patients for NSM.

### 11.7.1 *Size*

Size is considered by the plastic surgeon when considering reconstruction options, as well as by the breast surgeon when considering incision type. The skin envelope needs to be amenable to being filled by either an implant or a tissue flap. A cup, B cup, or C cup size breasts, for example, are easily reconstructed with either a tissue expander or autologous flap. Large C cup, D cup, or greater-size breasts pose a challenge when considering the choice of reconstruction techniques that allow the space below the skin envelope to be filled or reconstructed, and the NAC to be left in an acceptable position. A cup size breasts may be exceptionally suitable candidates for single-stage permanent implant procedures.

### 11.7.2 *Presence and Degree of Ptosis (Grade 1–3, Pseudoptosis)*

With severe ptosis, for example, optimal aesthetics may not be achievable after reconstruction without a free NAC transfer with skin reduction or a delayed skin-reduction procedure. The ideal breast shape/size for NSM with immediate reconstruction is an A cup, B cup, or C cup size. Breasts of size D cup or larger, or a significant degree of ptosis, do not preclude potential NSM. Techniques such as skin-reducing mastopexy, reducing mastectomy,[14] free nipple transfer, or a larger deep inferior epigastric perforator (DIEP), transverse rectus abdominis myocutaneous (TRAM), or extended latissimus dorsi flap will need to be considered/applied. A delayed skin reduction procedure, 3–4 months after NSM and reconstruction, is also an option.

## 11.8 Exclusionary Criteria

Inflammatory breast cancer, Paget's disease of the breast, or involvement of the NAC with cancer are definite exclusion criteria.

## 11.9 Preoperative Evaluation

### 11.9.1 *Clinical Breast Exam*

Size, shape, degree of ptosis, location of the NAC, areola size, skin condition, and prior scars are all noted. If the lesion is palpable at the level of the NAC, NSM is not an appropriate choice.

### 11.9.2 *Patient History*

Factors such as prior radiation therapy, BRCA status, and/or prior breast surgery are evaluated. If the patient has a history of radiation therapy for a previous cancer, the integrity and condition of the skin are evaluated as they would be for any mastectomy. A patient who is BRCA+ may also opt for a contralateral NSM as part of a risk-reduction strategy. A patient who has had a previous lumpectomy will be evaluated for utilizing the previous incision.

### 11.9.3 *Imaging*

A thorough evaluation of imaging is necessary in a preoperative evaluation. The distance of the lesion to the NAC should be measured. Published studies and case reviews outline utilization of ultrasound (US), mammogram, and/or MRI to aide in preoperative evaluation in predicting NAC involvement. Some advocate a radiographic distance of 1–5 cm; others utilize a lack of radiographically suspicious direct extension to the NAC.

Fukuma *et al.* utilize MRI magnification for optimal radiographic assessment of the NAC area and will core out the nipple even in the setting of radiographic evidence of potential NAC involvement. Currently, due to basic science research done on TDLUs, nipple anatomy, and realized rates of cancer in nipples, most surgeons rely on the permanent section of tissue immediately underlying the NAC for definitive management. This nipple core (tissue excised from immediately under the nipple) tissue analysis should be done routinely for all NSMs, including those performed in the prophylactic setting.

### 11.9.4 *Planning*

All patients undergoing a mastectomy can be considered potential candidates for NSM. The first criteria that need to be met are lack of clinical involvement of cancer with the NAC, no evidence of inflammatory breast cancer, and no evidence of Paget's disease. The next most important question is: "Can the plastic surgeon reconstruct a breast under the remaining skin envelope?" Location and type of incision alters both technical demand and the cosmetic outcome.

Work-up is identical to that for any type of mastectomy. Is the patient amenable to follow-up clinical exams? The patient must understand the possibility of NAC excision or conversion to areola-sparing if the final path assessment of the nipple core tissue is involved. Clinical follow-up exams are important for surveillance.

## 11.10 Plastic Reconstructive Surgery Considerations

The plastic surgeon involved will be able to assess breast size/shape/ptosis and decide whether to offer an aesthetically acceptable reconstruction, underneath the remaining skin envelope, in the event of NSM. Perhaps the key factor is the ability to provide a reconstructive option which leaves the NAC in a satisfactory position. Definitive implants, tissue expanders, autologous flaps, and delayed reconstruction have all been described as successful options. Some cases may require a larger autologous flap, a skin reduction with free nipple graft, or a delayed skin-reduction mastopexy. Patients may opt to undergo a contralateral symmetrizing procedure. All NSMs, including prophylactic, should have a nipple core specimen sent to pathology.

## 11.11 Comorbidities

The viability of the NAC is dependent on the surrounding flaps for blood supply. Comorbidities such as obesity, diabetes mellitus, significant peripheral vascular disease (PVD), smoking, and prior radiation may influence flap and the NAC viability. Very few articles on NSMs comment on the presence or absence of comorbidities. There is growing experience in performing NSMs in patients after a local recurrence from previous lumpectomy, and RT on women who are judged to have acceptable skin quality.

## 11.12 Intraoperative Technique

### 11.12.1 *Incision Planning*

Possible incisions that may be used for NSM include previous excision site, radial/lateral, radial/lateral with periareolar extension, radial 6 o'clock, Wise pattern, inframammary fold (IMF), axillary, trans-areola, and tumor site if in proximity to skin. For periareolar incisions, an incision limited to <30% of the circumference[13] is thought to be the least traumatic to the NAC and has been associated with reduced rates of epidermolysis and/or necrosis. Multiple incisions have been extensively reported as feasible.

### 11.12.2 *Spy Device*

This machine uses intraoperative fluorescent imaging (Figure 11.1) to allow for real-time assessment of blood flow of the skin. Some surgeons[15] report using the device to help optimize incision placement. In the patient represented in Figure 11.1, fluorescent imaging preoperatively changed the plan for the incision placement to a lower outer diagonal incision rather than a radial incision laterally, or an IMF incision. This allowed for preservation

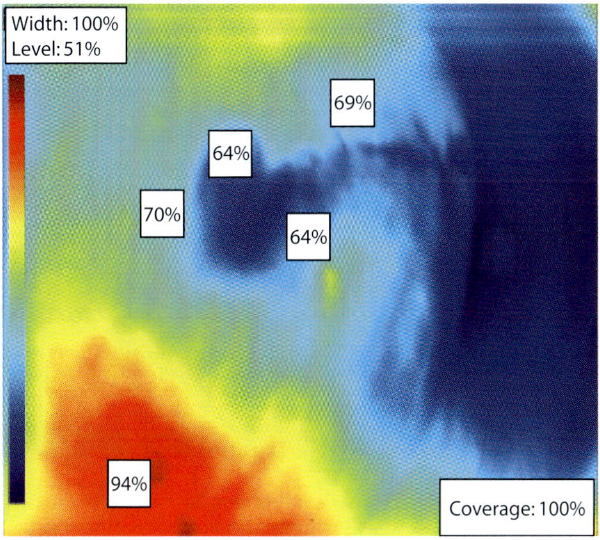


Figure 11.1. Fluorescent imaging preoperatively changed the plan for the incision placement to a lower outer diagonal incision.

of major feeding blood vessels that would have been traversed and likely injured in those areas. Postmastectomy fluorescent imaging confirmed excellent blood supply to all flaps.

### 11.12.3 *Inframammary Fold Incision*

An IMF incision may vary in length from patient to patient. This type of incision may be placed directly into the IMF line or slightly cephalad/caudad pending the anticipated final reconstructed result. Generally, this type of incision is well hidden post reconstruction. This incision is technically easier in the smaller breast (A cup or B cup). The distance from the IMF crease to the clavicle must also be reasonable enough to allow for instrument length and visualization in order to assure the removal of *all* breast tissue. If need be, a counteraxillary incision (the incision used in sentinel lymph node biopsy [SLNB]) may be helpful in dissecting the infraclavicular and upper outer quadrant regions. When utilizing an IMF or radial 6 o'clock incision, it is feasible to develop either the posterior or anterior plane first. Figure 11.2 represents a patient undergoing expansion of her tissue expanders (band-aid placement) with IMF line incisions that are well hidden.

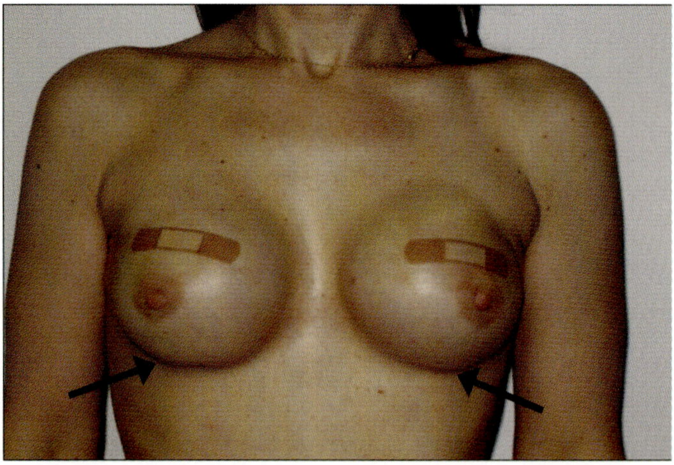

Figure 11.2. IMF line incision. Band-aids are used at the tissue expansion injection sites. The skin incisions are well hidden in the inframammary line (see arrows).

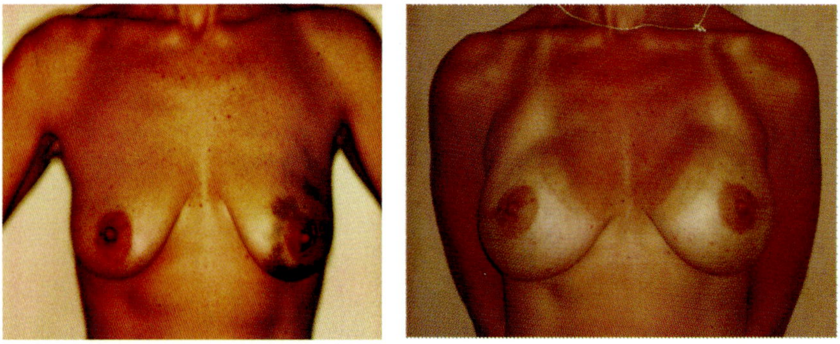

Figure 11.3. The left photograph shows the patient seen preoperatively. The right breast was ecchymotic after the core needle biopsy. The right photograph shows the patient in the postoperative period. Notice the lateral skin incisions bilaterally.

### 11.12.4 *Lateral Radial Incision*

A lateral radial incision (Figure 11.3) is perhaps the easiest incision type from a technical perspective. This type of incision can be performed either with or without extension into the areola, or periareolarly for increased exposure. This can generally be accomplished via a length of approximately 4 cm, or extended laterally as far as desired for increased exposure. Sentinel node biopsy and axillary node dissection can be easily performed via the same incision.

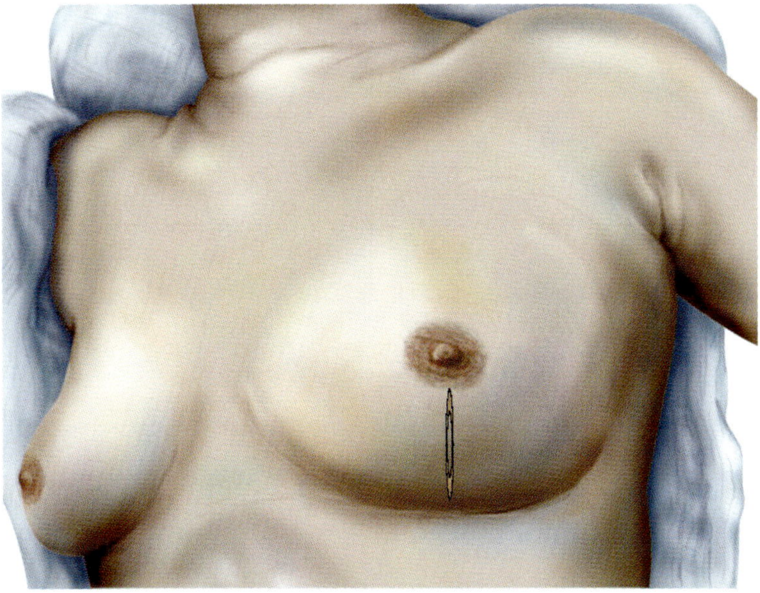

Figure 11.4. Radial 6 o'clock incision.

### 11.12.5 *Radial 6 O'clock Incision*

A radial 6 o'clock incision (Figure 11.4) also results in superior cosmetic outcome status after reconstruction as the incision is well hidden. This incision can be extended into the areola if need be. This incision, as well as an IMF incision, can be technically challenging with either a large or a ptotic breast. The addition of a short axillary incision (utilized for SLNB) may be utilized in facilitating upper-pole dissection.

### 11.12.6 *Previous Lumpectomy Scar Incision*

A previous lumpectomy site scar (Figure 11.5) can be utilized via an elliptical excision of the scar. Exposure can be increased by making a counter axillary incision if needed.

### 11.12.7 *Transareolar Incision*

Though infrequently utilized, this type of incision (Figure 11.6) has also been described as providing sufficient exposure.

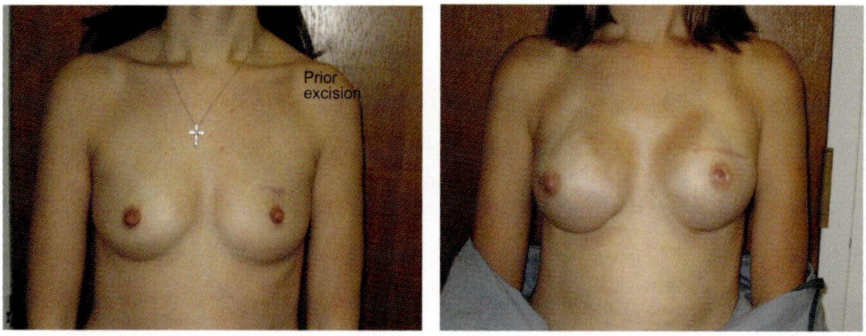


Figure 11.5. Previous lumpectomy scar incision. The left photograph is a preoperative view of a patient with a left breast lumpectomy scar that will be excised and used for completion of the mastectomy. The right photograph shows the same patient postoperatively. The right mastectomy was performed through a lateral radial incision.

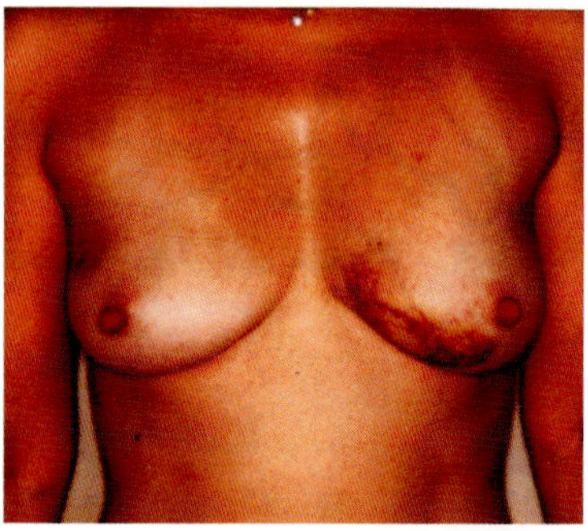

(a)

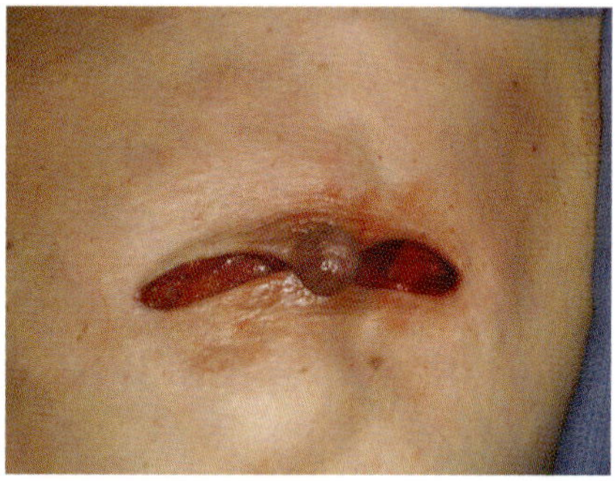

(b)

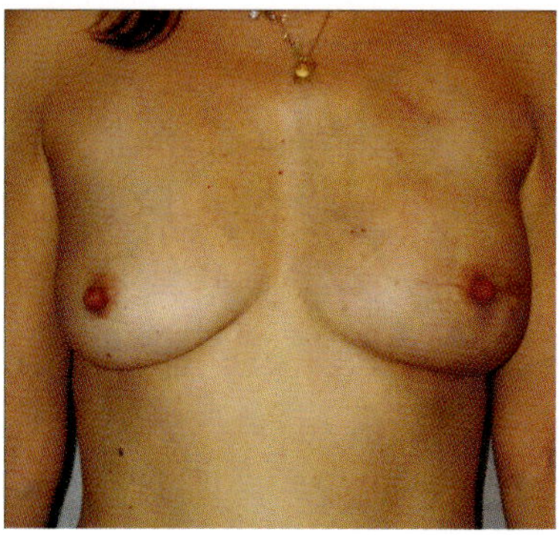

(c)

Figure 11.6. Transareolar incision. (a) Preoperative view of the patient; (b) Intraoperative view of the incision after removal of the breast. The nipple is part of the upper flap; (c) The postoperative result. The right breast was not operated on.

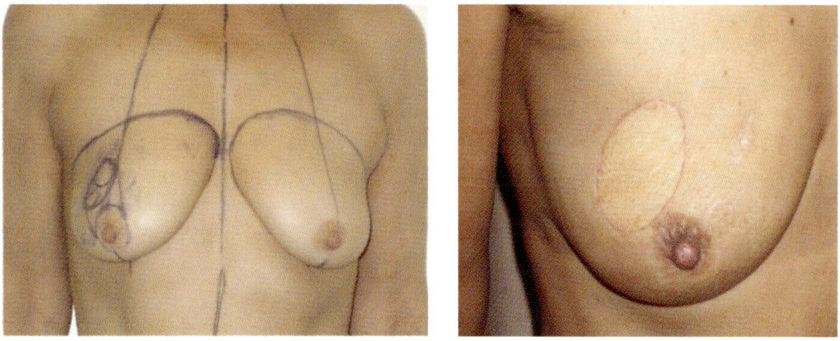

Figure 11.7. Tumor site incision and reconstruction with a DIEP flap. Note how the abdominal skin was limited to cover the area of the breast skin excised with the mastectomy.

### 11.12.8 *Tumor Site Incision*

An incision may be made directly overlying a superficial tumor (Figure 11.7). Sentinel node biopsy and axillary node dissection may be performed through prior lumpectomy incisions when located in the upper outer quadrant of the breast. The patient presented in Figure 11.7 had an immediate reconstruction with a DIEP flap.

## 11.13 Endoscopy

Performing NSM via endoscopic technique has been utilized by our Japanese colleagues for many years with excellent cosmetic and oncologic results. A recently published article[16] outlines a case series of 89 mastectomies performed for breast cancer in patients without skin or nipple involvement. They reported a follow-up period of 52 months demonstrating distant recurrence in nine patients, no local recurrences, and no nipple involvement. They utilized a 3-cm axillary incision, which was extended to 5 cm if the SLNB was found to be positive and an axillary lymph node dissection was performed. They note that this technique is accomplished with ease among women with small (A cup size) non-ptotic breasts. The ability to perform NSM with this technique has significant cultural significance in that it allows women to participate in traditional public bath or steam room/sauna use with only trace evidence of having ever had surgery.

### 11.13.1 *Endoscopic Technique*

The posterior dissection between the breast and the pectoralis major muscle is completed as much as possible under direct visualization. A 30-degree scope is used for continuing the posterior dissection endoscopically using either an ultraretractor and/or bipolar scissors. On completion of posterior dissection, they recommend a periareolar incision (less than one-half of the circumference). They then raise the first 2 cm of the subdermal skin flaps under direct visualization. Next, a bladeless tracer is utilized to create parallel tunnels at 2-cm intervals within the subdermal plane. They then insert a zero-degree scope and cut the septa with bipolar scissors under direct visualization. Next, they core the nipple and send the tissue immediately under the NAC as a separate specimen.

### 11.13.2 *Accessing SLNB*

SLNB can often be performed through the same incision utilized for the NSM. If this is not feasible, a separate axillary incision can be made with ease. When utilizing periareolar blue dye for sentinel node mapping, it is not unusual to note discoloration of the skin, which may make it difficult to assess the intraoperative viability of the NAC. Many surgeons only use radioisotope to avoid this issue.

### 11.13.3 *Dissection*

Dissection can be accomplished either through electrocautery or through tumescent injection with sharp dissection. Dissecting between the subdermal and subcutaneous plane is optimal for flap dissection. When utilizing tumescent solution, inject it into the subcutaneous space in a fanning/radial pattern. The area under the NAC can also be infiltrated in attempts to aid in hemostasis during inframammary NAC dissection. Sharp dissection then proceeds in between the subdermal and subcutaneous space. If electrocautery is utilized to raise the flaps, it is recommended to switch to sharp dissection (knife or metz) for the subareolar tissue/nipple core in order to limit trauma to the NAC. Light (in the form of lighted retractors or a light map on the retractor) will significantly aid this process.

### 11.13.4 *Coring*

Within the literature, the term "coring" has become synonymous with the thoughtful, active removal of all breast tissue underlying the NAC. This can be done safely by everting the NAC over the second finger of the nondominant hand and utilizing sharp dissection (using either a metz or scalpel) to excise all the tissue underlying the dermis (Figure 11.8). This breast tissue is the nipple core tissue sample that is sent separately for pathology analysis. This tissue can be sent for frozen section or permanent pathology. The

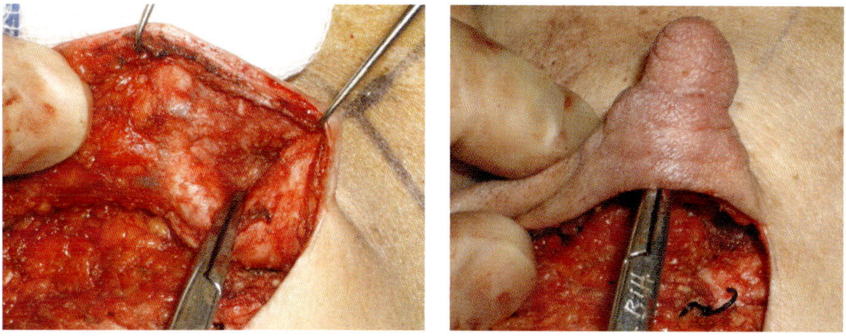

Figure 11.8. Everting the NAC over the second finger of the non-dominant hand and utilizing sharp dissection to excise all the tissue underlying the dermis.

patient must be educated preoperatively that if this tissue comes back positive for cancer at any time, the NAC or nipple will be removed (whether intraoperatively with a frozen section or in the office upon final pathology evaluation). The NAC can be excised as an office procedure. Patients with nipple-core involvement can be converted to an areola-sparing mastectomy with delayed nipple reconstruction. Nipple involvement by invasive carcinoma or DCIS has been identified by analysis of the retroareolar margin with a sensitivity of 0.8 and a negative predictive value of 0.96.[9]

## 11.14 Additional Technical Notes

If suspicion arises in the OR of possible close skin margin, place a nylon stitch in both the skin and the specimen directly underlying to mark the spot. If that specimen comes back with positive anterior margins, you will already have the skin marked for easy local excision, which can be done in the office at a later time after flap and NAC healing are complete. Pre-NSM devascularization of the NAC is a technique utilized by some. The premise is to make a periareolar incision "several weeks" preoperatively in efforts to enhance the blood supply after the NSM. Jensen *et al.*[17] described an incidence rate of 0% nipple necrosis when patients underwent a pre-NSM surgical delay procedure in the setting of increased risk of nipple necrosis.

## 11.15 Intraoperative Radiation with Electrons (ELIOT)

ELIOT has been extensively described as a potential adjuvant technique to add to NSMs.[14,18–20] These studies describe an intraoperative RT with electrons of 16 Gy in one single fraction delivered to the NAC with lead and aluminum disk protection of the chest wall and pectoralis muscle. Immediate reconstruction generally entailed a definitive prosthesis, a tissue expander, or, less commonly, a tissue flap. The majority of the published work reports a 5-year follow-up of no significant differences noted between patients receiving ELIOT (800 patients) versus delayed radiation (201 patients). No noticeable differences were noticed in complication rates or rates of relapse (0.9% per year, always at the original tumor site, and never at the NAC) between patient or tumor features.[19,20] Surgical technique in these series varies from the standard NSM. Flaps were elevated in the subdermal plane, but the infra-areolar tissue was dealt with differently. The published work did report leaving a "thin layer" of glandular tissue below the NAC to preserve blood supply.[19] Under this preserved tissue, a small section of inframammary NAC tissue was excised for immediate frozen section; if the frozen section was positive, an additional layer of inframammary NAC tissue was removed for frozen section. If the second frozen section was positive, the NAC was excised.[19] Nevertheless, no recurrence was noted to occur at the level of the NAC.[14,18–20] Dr Jean Y. Petit has reported that he will be starting a trial comparing NSM with or without intraoperatve radiation therapy.[21] It is his belief that ELIOT is not required for all patients.

## 11.16 Outcomes

### 11.16.1 *Viability*

The viability of both flaps and the NAC are of utmost interest. Perhaps the most significant factor predicting flap and NAC viability is surgical technique. Careful and gentle handling and/or retracting of both flaps and the NAC are important. Full-thickness NAC necrosis, necessitating excision, has been reported in $\leq$10% of reported cases.[2,14,18,22,23] If epidermolysis (sloughing) of the NAC does occur, it will typically resolve on its own. If it achieves a level of full-thickness necrosis and there is risk of implant infection, the NAC should be excised. If excision is necessary, it can generally be done in the office. The patient should always be counseled preoperatively of this possibility.

### 11.16.2 *Sensation*

Innervation of the NAC is derived from the anterior and lateral cutaneous branches of the second through fourth intercostal nerves. Most literature reports loss of nipple sensation status after NSM; some degree of nipple sensation has been reported to be preserved in 15%–75% of reported cases.[14,23,24] Patients should be counseled that they are most likely to have no postoperative nipple sensation.

### 11.16.3 *Aesthetics*

Women report feeling "less mutilated"[20,23] when undergoing NSM. They have also used terminology such as "psychological calmness"; "wholeness"; and "more natural appearing."[23] Body-image perception, patient satisfaction, and psychological adjustment have also been noted to be superior with NSM.[20] Objective cosmetic outcomes and patient satisfaction have been noted to be superior to a non-NSM and equal to BCT.[19]

### 11.16.4 *Recurrence Rates*

Recurrence should be monitored by clinical exam as after any type of mastectomy. Most reports in the literature refer to a rate of recurrence of <10% comparable to TM or BCT with radiation therapy (RT) (Table 11.2). There are only anecdotal, isolated cases of nipple recurrence at the level of the nipple. The cumulative world experience both reported in the literature and anecdotally at scientific symposiums leads us to believe that the absolute risk of nipple recurrence is extremely small. With this remote risk of recurrence, management of oncologic consequences should be minimal with the excision of the nipple. It should also be very easy to detect should it occur.

In a case series of 579 NSMs with IORT (ELIOT),[2] no difference was found in the local recurrence rate according to patients or tumor features; recurrences were noted in the tumor bed but never in the NAC. In a study of 1,001 patients undergoing NSM, a comparison of ELIOT (800 patients) with delayed RT (201 patients) showed no significant difference in outcomes, including recurrence.[14]

Editorial Comment

In the January 2012 issue of *Annals of Oncology* (PMID: 22231025), Petit JY *et al.* published their update of the European Institute of Oncology (EIO) experience with NSM and ELIOT on 772 invasive cancers and 162 intra-epithelial neoplasias. The median follow-up was 50 months. The in-breast and NAC local recurrence rates for invasive cancer were 3.6% and 0.8%, respectively. More concerning are the in-breast and NAC recurrence rates for DCIS, which were 4.9% and 2.9%, respectively. These rates of recurrence are significantly higher than previously reported with short-term follow-up.

The mastectomy technique used at the EIO differs from the one reported in this chapter. The editor would like to caution surgeons on the importance of long-term follow-up with these new endeavors. The editor recommends adherence to strict selection criteria, adherence to safe oncologic techniques of mastectomy, and appropriate training. I also recommend reporting all NSM cases to local or national registries in order to maintain tracking of long-term results.

### 11.16.5 *Prophylactic NSM*

No evidence of carcinoma or DCIS in prophylactic mastectomy nipples has been found. The Mayo series may also be considered in prophylactic NSMs.

## 11.17 Clinical Pearls

### 11.17.1 *What Is the Learning Curve?*

When completing your first NSM, it is important to plan an incision that will result in easy accessibility to all breast tissue (the radial/lateral incision is the easiest approach to start); one should also have the appropriate instruments, pay special attention not to place too much tension on the flaps while dissecting, and remove all tissue underlying the NAC. It is critically important that the traditional anatomical landmarks used to designate complete removal of the breast be adhered to in order to insure that residual breast tissue is not left behind.

### 11.17.2 *What Special Instruments Are Required?*

Exposure is typically less extensive when performing NSM. Lighted retractors or a light map added to the retractors, is extremely helpful. A Bovie extension and/or long-face lift scissors are also often necessary.

## 11.18 Summary and Conclusions

### 11.18.1 *Unresolved Issues Postmastectomy*

NSM is a type of mastectomy that is increasingly being performed to date. Recurrence rates have been consistently as low as or lower than those of traditional mastectomies. Patients benefit from the overall improved cosmesis and in not having to lose the NAC (or nipple with an areola-sparing procedure) unnecessarily. Current metrics are evolving. The NSM

Registry of the American Society of Breast Surgeons will provide outcome measures (local recurrence, locoregional recurrence, and overall survival), as well as delineated metrics, surgical technique, and patient characteristics, via a prospective registry. Surgeons are currently relying more on the inframammary NAC tissue specimen to determine the fate of the nipple. This is a technically demanding procedure. To ensure complete removal of all breast tissue through limited incisions requires training and mentorship. We believe that this is extremely worthwhile for patients in terms of quality of life and aesthetic appearance. For appropriately selected patients, it is oncologically safe. Our knowledge base will continue to expand as large datasets are developed through the NSM Registry of the American Society of Breast Surgeons.

## References


1. Didier F, Radice D, Gandini S, *et al.* (2009) Does nipple preservation in mastectomy improve satisfaction with cosmetic results, psychological adjustment, body image and sexuality? *Breast Cancer Res Treat* 118(3): 623–633.
2. Ueda S, Tamaki Y, Yano K, *et al.* (2008) Cosmetic outcome and patient satisfaction after skin-sparing mastectomy for breast cancer with immediate reconstruction of the breast. *Surgery* 143(3):414–425.
3. Yueh JH, Houlihan MJ, Slavin SA, *et al.* (2009) Nipple-sparing mastectomy: Evaluation of patient satisfaction, aesthetic results, and sensation. *Ann Plast Surg* 62(5):586–590.
4. Petit JY, Veronesi U, Orecchia R, *et al.* (2007) The nipple sparing mastectomy: A 5-year experience at the European Institute of Oncology of Milan. *Br Can Res* 9:510.
5. Hartmann LC, Schaid DJ, Woods JE, *et al.* (1999) Efficacy of bilateral prophylactic mastectomy in women with a family history of breast cancer. *N Engl J Med* 340(2):77–84.
6. Rusby JE, Brachtel EF, Michaelson JS, *et al.* (2007) Breast duct anatomy in the human nipple: Three-dimensional patterns and clinical implications. *Breast Cancer Res Treat* 106(2):171–179.
7. Banerjee A, Gupta S, Bhattacharya N. (2008) Preservation of nipple-areola complex in breast cancer — A clinicopathological assessment. *J Plast Reconstr Aesthet Surg* 61(10):1195–1198.
8. Simmons RM, Brennan M, Christos P, King V, Osborne M. (2002) Analysis of nipple/areolar involvement with mastectomy: can the areola be preserved? *Ann Surg Oncol* 9(2):165–168.
9. Brachtel EF, Rusby JE, Michaelson JS, *et al.* (2009) Occult nipple involvement in breast cancer: Clinicopathologic findings in 316 consecutive mastectomy specimens. *J Clin Oncol* 27(30):4948–4954.
10. Rusby JE, Brachtel EF, Othus M, *et al.* (2008) Development and validation of a model predictive of occult nipple involvement in women undergoing mastectomy. *Br J Surg* 95(11):1356–1361.

11. Fukuma E (2011) Personal correspondence, Eisuke Fukuma, MD, Breast Center, Kameda Medical Center, 929 Higashi-Cho, Kamogawa, Chiba 296-8602, Japan.
12. Bloom S, Morrow M (2010) A clinical oncologic perspective on breast magnetic resonance imaging. *Magn Reson Imaging Clin N Am* 18(2):277–294, ix.
13. Loewen MJ, Jennings JA, Sherman SR, *et al.* (2008) Mammographic distance as a predictor of nipple-areola complex involvement in breast cancer. *Am J Surg* 195(3):391–394; discussion 4–5.
14. Rusby JE, Gui GP. (2010) Nipple-sparing mastectomy in women with large or ptotic breasts. *J Plast Reconstr Aesthet Surg* 63(10):e754–755.
15. Bailey L. (2011) Personal correspondence, Lisa Bailey MD, Medical Director, Carol Ann Read Breast Health Center, Oakland, CA 94609, USA.
16. Sakamoto N, Fukuma E, Higa K, *et al.* (2009) Early results of an endoscopic nipple-sparing mastectomy for breast cancer. *Ann Surg Oncol* 16(12):3406–3413.
17. Jensen JA, Orringer JS, Giuliano AE. (2011) Nipple-sparing mastectomy in 99 patients with a mean follow-up of 5 years. *Ann Surg Oncol* 18(6):1665–1670.
18. Petit JY, Veronesi U, Luini A, *et al.* (2005) When mastectomy becomes inevitable: The nipple-sparing approach. *Breast* 14(6):527–531.
19. Petit JY, Veronesi U, Orecchia R, *et al.* (2009) Nipple sparing mastectomy with nipple areola intraoperative radiotherapy: One thousand and one cases of a five years experience at the European Institute of Oncology of Milan (EIO). *Breast Cancer Res Treat* 117(2):333–338.
20. Petit JY, Veronesi U, Rey P, *et al.* (2009) Nipple-sparing mastectomy: Risk of nipple-areolar recurrences in a series of 579 cases. *Breast Cancer Res Treat* 114(1):97–101.
21. Petit JY. (2011) Personal correspondence, Jean Y. Petit, MD, Division of Plastic Surgery, European Institute of Oncology, Via Ripamonti, 435, 20141 Milano, Italy.
22. Regolo L, Ballardini B, Gallarotti E, *et al.* (2008) Nipple sparing mastectomy: An innovative skin incision for an alternative approach. *Breast* 17(1):8–11.
23. Sookhan N, Boughey JC, Walsh MF, Degnim AC. (2008) Nipple-sparing mastectomy — Initial experience at a tertiary center. *Am J Surg* 196(4): 575–577.
24. Wijayanayagam A, Kumar AS, Foster RD, Esserman LJ. (2008) Optimizing the total skin — Sparing mastectomy. *Arch Surg* 143(1):38–45; discussion.
25. Voltura AM, Tsangaris TN, Rosson GD, *et al.* (2008) Nipple-sparing mastectomy: Critical assessment of 51 procedures and implications for selection criteria. *Ann Surg Oncol* 15(12):3396–3401.
26. Crowe JP, Jr., Kim JA, Yetman R, *et al.* (2004) Nipple-sparing mastectomy: Technique and results of 54 procedures. *Arch Surg* 139(2):148–150.
27. Crowe JP, Patrick RJ, Yetman RJ, Djohan R. (2008) Nipple-sparing mastectomy update: One hundred forty-nine procedures and clinical outcomes. *Arch Surg* 143(11):1106–1110; discussion 10.

28. Sacchini V, Pinotti JA, Barros AC, *et al.* (2006) Nipple-sparing mastectomy for breast cancer and risk reduction: Oncologic or technical problem? *J Am Coll Surg* 203(5):704–714.
29. Lagios MD, Gates EA, Westdahl PR, *et al.* (1979) A guide to the frequency of nipple involvement in breast cancer. A study of 149 consecutive mastectomies using a serial subgross and correlated radiographic technique. *Am J Surg* 138(1):135–142.
30. Garwood ER, Moore D, Ewing C, *et al.* (2009) Total skin-sparing mastectomy: Complications and local recurrence rates in 2 cohorts of patients. *Ann Surg* 249(1):26–32.
31. Nahabedian MY, Tsangaris TN. (2006) Breast reconstruction following subcutaneous mastectomy for cancer: A critical appraisal of the nipple-areola complex. *Plast Reconstr Surg* 117(4):1083–1090.
32. Gerber B, Krause A, Dieterich M, *et al.* (2009) The oncological safety of skin sparing mastectomy with conservation of the nipple-areola complex and autologous reconstruction: An extended follow-up study. *Ann Surg* 249(3):461–468.

# Chapter 12

# RADIATION THERAPY

Robert R. Kuske, Jr.
*Arizona Oncology Services Cancer Research Foundation*
*Scottsdale, AZ 85260, USA*

## 12.1 Background

Lumpectomy and axillary node sampling (for invasive cancers), followed by breast radiotherapy (RT), has been the standard for local therapy of most stage Tis, T1, T2, N0, and N1 breast cancers since the late 1980s.[1] Like mastectomy, breast RT aims to cover the whole breast tissue and, when indicated, the surrounding lymphatics. Because the RT fields encompass a large volume of tissue, and because they enter and exit through the skin, a dose-limiting organ, the dose is typically divided into relatively small daily fractions over 6–7 weeks to reduce side effects and late fibrosis. Landmark single-institution prospective clinical trials[2,3] and a phase II cooperative group trial, Radiation Therapy Oncology Group (RTOG) 95-17,[4,5] have provided the impetus for a 5-day partial breast irradiation (PBI) alternative to the conventional whole breast irradiation (WBI) of 6–7 weeks. PBI has become an increasingly popular option, with low toxicity and excellent cosmetic outcomes.[6]

Paralleling the success and growth rate of PBI, oncoplastic surgery is becoming an increasingly popular method of breast-conserving surgery (BCS). Oncoplastic surgery uses the best principles of plastic and reconstructive surgery, melded with optimal cancer surgery techniques of removal of the tumor with generous margins of normal tissue, frequently involving quadrantectomy.[7] The resulting surgical scars are longer and usually bilateral, but the size, shape, symmetry, and overall cosmetic outcomes tend to be excellent.[8]

Many breast specialists would likely appreciate the opportunity to merge the 2 increasingly popular breast cancer local therapies of PBI and oncoplastic surgery.

The problem to be overcome, however, is that oncoplastic surgery closes the lumpectomy cavity so that no seroma develops, eliminating the usual target for PBI. To perform targeted RT, most techniques require a cavity or seroma. It is impossible to place a balloon catheter or a multistrut hybrid brachytherapy device without a space in the breast for the intracavitary catheter to reside. Interstitial brachytherapy does not require a lumpectomy cavity, but it too requires target volume delineation, which is usually obliterated by oncoplastic surgery. Taking these factors into consideration, we find that these 2 emerging innovative surgical and RT methodologies — PBI and oncoplastic surgery — are not necessarily incompatible.

## 12.2 Oncoplastic Surgery and 5-Day Interstitial Brachytherapy

In our practice, we prospectively treat selected women with the following techniques in response to an observed increase in the number of women pursing oncoplastic surgery with Tis, T1, T2, N0, N1 (1–3 positive nodes without extracapsular-nodal extension)[9,10]:

- A wide local excision or quadrantectomy is performed with clear margins by at least 1 mm, and usually much wider with sentinel node mapping/biopsy if the tumor was invasive.
- At least 6 surgical clips are placed prior to moving tissue around and closing the cavity (superior, inferior, medial, lateral, superficial, deep, and another where the surgeon thinks the margin is closest).
- Oncoplastic tissue manipulation to close the cavity and shape the breast, leaving the clips attached to the original cavity wall, with the ultimate location of the clips ending up in various new locations within the breast.
- A radiation oncology consultation 2–4 weeks after surgery with the pathology report available.
- Postlumpectomy mammography in radiology (Figure 12.1) and computed tomography (CT) of the breast in radiation oncology to evaluate where the clips ended up.
- Interdisciplinary deliberation regarding the patient's candidacy for PBI.
- If approved, the patient is scheduled for image-guided insertion of interstitial brachytherapy catheters at the Arizona Breast Cancer Specialists facility in Arizona.
- On the procedure day, the patient is positioned supine on the CT table with arms extended over the head, prepped, and draped in sterile fashion.

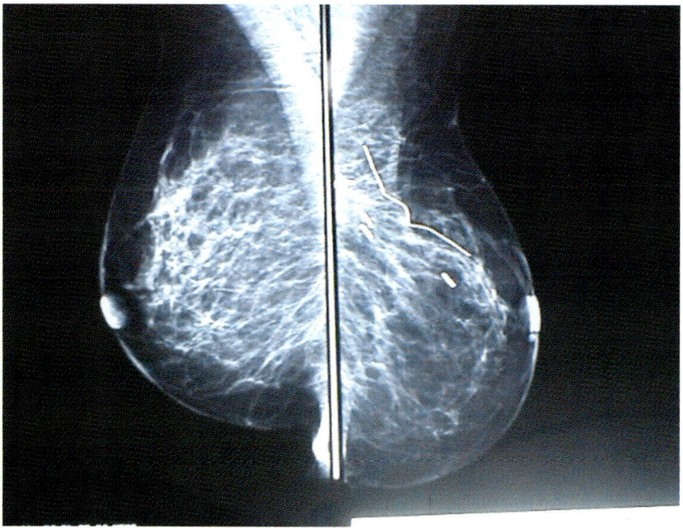

Figure 12.1. Mammography after oncoplastic surgery before accelerated PBI. The breast exhibits a wire taped to the skin over the quadrantectomy skin incision scar. The surgical clips are noted to extend over the entire quadrant; they provide a clear target for image-guided interstitial brachytherapy catheter insertion.

- The involved breast is massaged and lifted up and away from the chest wall, while the template is attached with moderate compression.
- Using 27G and 25G needles, and dilute buffered local anesthetic, 3 pathways are locally anesthetized, and 3 anchoring 5F brachytherapy needles, are inserted through pre-drilled holes in the template to prevent slippage.
- A CT (with 2.5 mm slices) is obtained through the ipsilateral breast and with the quadrentectomy scar wired.
- The radiation oncologist locates all 6 clips and any postoperative scar on the CT that is associated with the original lumpectomy cavity, and contours the "lumpectomy" target volume on a 3-dimensional computerized treatment planning system (3dTPS) (Figure 12.2).
- The 3dTPS increases the target volume by 2 cm in all dimensions, creating a planning treatment volume (PTV) (Figure 12.2).
- The dosimetrist or medical physicist pulls the PTV 5 mm from the skin and up to the pectoralis fascia, creating the PTV-eval.
- The 3dTPS rotates the computer rendition of the breast in 3-dimensional space until the holes in the front and back templates are perfectly aligned. The PTV-eval is displayed, revealing which holes need to be filled with brachytherapy needles to cover the grown target volume but avoid the pleura (Figure 12.2).

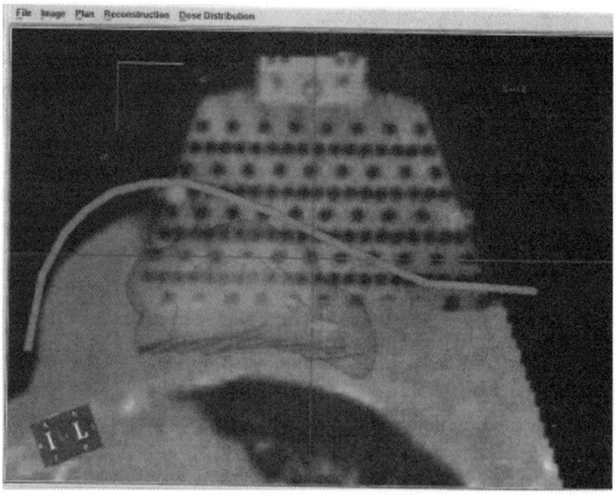

Figure 12.2. A polyphenlylsulfone template is attached to the ipsilateral breast with moderate compression. The template has pre-drilled holes for the insertion of brachytherapy needles that are replaced eventually by plastic catheters with buttons on each end to prevent slippage. Note the inner darker blue volume that correlates to the clips placed at the periphery of the cavity after the lumpectomy but before tissue movement and closure of the cavity. The outer lighter blue volume represents a 2 cm growth of the clip volume and is the target volume for catheter coverage.

- Diluted local anesthetic mixture with epinephrine is injected down each planned pathway through the template holes. This procedure is typically painless and bloodless.
- 5F brachytherapy needles are quickly inserted through the template with 1.5 cm between needles and 2 cm between rows, for an average of 24 needles.
- The template is disassembled and removed, leaving the needles in the breast.
- The thin end of the plastic 6F Comfort catheters is inserted into each needle and pulled through the breast, replacing the needle. The needle is then discarded (Figure 12.3).
- Later that day or the following day, after the swelling has subsided, another CT is obtained for treatment planning, source-dwell–position selection, and dose calculation.
- In dosimetry, we insist on 95% dose coverage of at least 95% of PTV-eval. The skin dose never exceeds the prescription dose. The 150% isodose curves between catheters can kiss but not coalesce (Figure 12.4). The dose homogeneity index (DHI) should be in the 80% to 85% range.
- Allowing a day for the physics team to perfect the dosimetry and sculpt the dose cloud, brachytherapy starts on the second working day after the procedure.

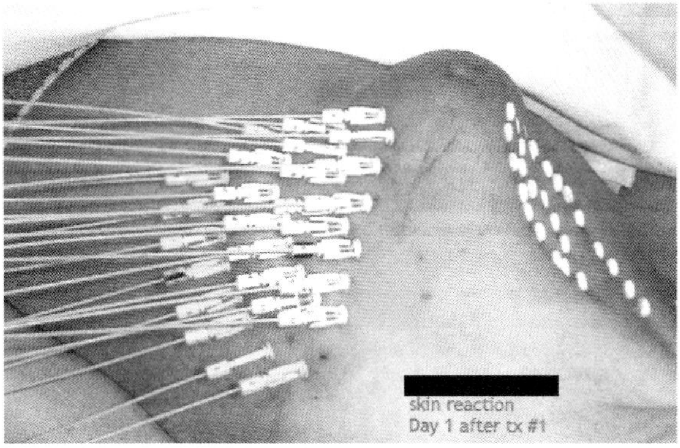


Figure 12.3. Photograph of the left breast after the first of 10 brachytherapy fractions with 26 plastic catheters in place that generously cover the target volume. To cover this volume after a quadrantectomy requires a myriad of catheters, but the insertion is painless and bloodless under local anesthetic with the patient awake.

- Using a high dose-rate remote afterloader, an iridium-192 seed ($3 \times 1$ mm) is run down each catheter, stopping at 5 mm intervals, with the dwell time determining the dose delivery to the target issue. With an average of 10–12 dwell positions in each catheter, there are approximately 250 stopping points of the radioactive seed for each treatment, providing an opportunity to precisely sculpt the dose cloud by varying the dwell times at each position.
- 34 Gray is given in 10 fractions over 5 treatment days, with at least 6 hours between fractions.
- After the tenth interstitial brachytherapy, the button on one side of each catheter is snipped, and all catheters are removed simultaneously with very little discomfort and no anesthesia.
- Prophylactic antibiotics are not used, but approximately 15% of patients may need antibiotic treatment for erythema, fever, chills, or other symptoms.
- The patient is seen a week after catheter removal to evaluate healing and check for delayed infection.
- The first follow-up mammography is 6 months after the final brachytherapy date, with the treated breast being imaged every 6 months for 2 years, and annually thereafter. Cosmetic outcome in one of Dr. Silverstein's patients at 6 months follow-up after image-guided brachytherapy is shown in Figure 12.5.

Our experience with interstitial brachytherapy and with over 1,600 treated patients has shown recurrence rates of 4% at 5 years and 5% at 7 years.[2,11] William Beaumont Hospital in Michigan reported a matched

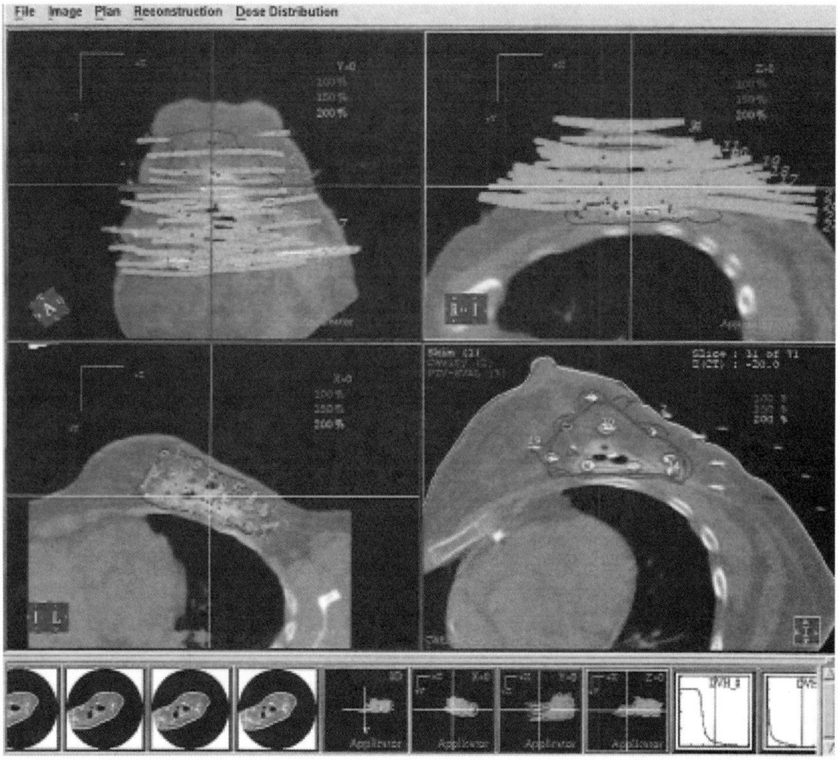


Figure 12.4. Surgical clips delineate the edges of the original lumpectomy cavity before oncoplastic movement of tissue to close the cavity. A CT is obtained in the radiation oncology department with a special brachytherapy template attached. The 3-dimensional computerized treatment planning system (3dTPS) demonstrates the surgical clips, contoured on each CT-slice, that are rendered on a 3-dimensional view with the front and back templates aligned. The top left and right computer renditions show the catheters in coronal and sagittal views. The bottom left view displays the highly conformal dose distribution lines (100% red, 150% green, and 200% yellow). The bottom right view shows a transverse CT slice through the nipple with remnants of the surgical cavity still evident after oncoplastic surgery, and with catheter coverage evident and the dosimetry displayed. Please note that the heart/coronary artery dose with traditional tangential external radiation fields would have been high, minimized by accelerated PBI.

pair analysis (PBI versus WBI) at 10 years follow-up with no significant difference in local recurrence, survival, or cosmesis.[12] The RTOG 95–17 results with multi-institution interstitial brachytherapy show a 5% recurrence rate of 5 years.[4] The prospective randomized phase III Hungarian trial with interstitial brachytherapy versus WBI shows equivalent local control but a trend toward better cosmetic outcome with brachytherapy.[13] Five ongoing

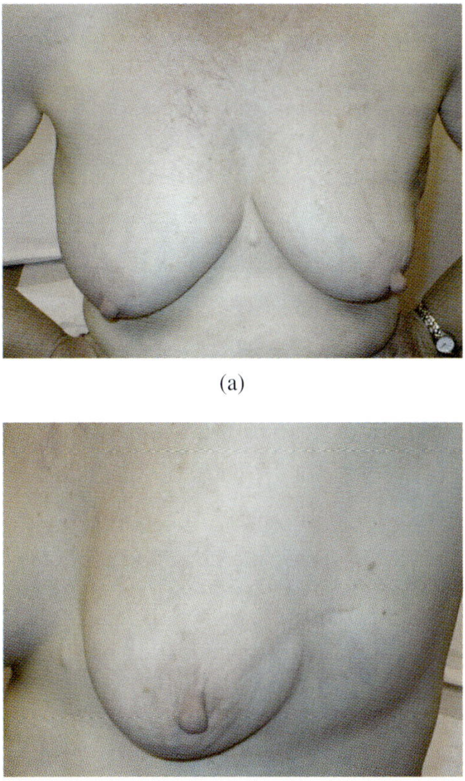

(a)

(b)

Figure 12.5. The cosmetic outcome in a patient 6 months after interstitial brachytherapy following breast-conserving oncoplastic surgery.

randomized trials, including National Surgical Adjuvant Breast and Bowel Project (NSABP)-B39, should shed considerable light on PBI as a 5-day alternative to conventional 6–7 week WBI, especially in certain high-risk subsets.

Unfortunately, patients undergoing oncoplastic lumpectomy/quadrantectomy with tissue movement to obliterate the cavity have not been included in the above clinical trials. Our experience so far is at its inception, with only 12 treated patients. There have been no local recurrences at a median follow-up of 3 years. All 12 have had good or excellent cosmetic outcomes without telangiectosia, fat necrosis, or significant fibrosis. The future success of brachytherapy after oncoplastic surgery will be prospective clinical trials. Eventually, the number of surgeons who have learned these techniques will reach a critical mass where such studies are feasible. However, radiation oncologists must likewise learn interstitial brachytherapy, which may prove to be a major bottleneck.

## 12.3 Oncoplastic Surgery with 3-Dimensional Conformal PBI

The other major current PBI technique that does not necessarily depend on a cavity/seroma for RT delivery is external-beam 3-dimensional conformal PBI.[14] Indeed, this PBI technique has been chosen by 75% of all participants in the ongoing NSABP-B39 clinical trial who were randomized to PBI.

Similar to the above discussion regarding target volume delineation with interstitial brachytherapy, the surgeon must leave clips so that there is a target for the radiation. The clips should be placed after the lumpectomy or quadrantectomy, but before tissue mobilization and closure of the cavity. The clips should be placed at the superior, inferior, medial, lateral, superficial, and deep extent of the lumpectomy edges. An extra clip where the surgeon deems the closest margin is located can also be helpful.

After tissue mobilization and movement to close the lumpectomy cavity and shape the breast, note that the clips will ultimately be widely located. Because of this wide clip separation, defining the target volume can be challenging. The PTV-eval treatment volume features a 2.5-cm growth beyond the clips. Multiple beams are tightly collimated with custom blocking to the shape of the PTV-eval. Our technique, called the "helicopter rotor" technique, employs 4 non-coplanar beams. The treatment couch is rotated 20 degrees off the usual medial and lateral tangential fields and then bent backward by 5 degrees to resemble the angles of a helicopter rotor. The fields are then blocked to conform to the shape of the PTV-eval at that angle. There are no published data using the technique after oncoplastic surgery.

## 12.4 Intraoperative Radiotherapy During Oncoplastic Surgery

Another feasible approach to PBI in conjunction with oncoplastic surgery is intraoperative radiotherapy (IORT). Current methods include electron beam, intrabeam, balloon catheters, and catheter-based applicators such as the 2–10 channel HAM applicator. After the lumpectomy/quadrantectomy and before tissue mobilization to close the cavity, a single fraction of 21 Gray is delivered using electron beam. Lead shielding is placed in front of the chest wall behind the breast tissue to avoid electron penetration into the lung and subsequent increase in risk of radiation pneumonitis.

Quality assurance with this technique requires definition. Currently, the volume of tissue beyond the cavity wall that is treated is nebulous and varies from investigator to investigator. After the electron beam treatment, oncoplastic closure of the cavity and shaping of the breast are immediately performed. The advantages of this technique include completion of all local therapy in 1 day, and skin hooks holding the skin away from the beam so the skin dose is minimized. Potential issues are the lack of a pathology report before RT to indicate that the patient is a candidate for PBI, potential wound-healing problems, and under-treatment of breast tissue clinging to the skin being retracted during electron beam delivery. A large randomized Italian trial of intraoperative electrons after lumpectomy is complete but not yet reported. There are no data regarding this technique in association with oncoplastic surgery.

Intrabeam delivers soft X-rays using a metal ball that is inserted into the lumpectomy cavity during the surgery, but before tissue mobilization, cavity closure, and breast shaping. The soft X-rays do not penetrate deeply into tissue, so the therapeutic dose only reaches 2 mm beyond the surgical edge. The dose at 1 cm beyond the cavity is homeopathic, and is negligible at 2 cm.

Balloon catheters such as the Axxent Balloon Applicator (XOFT, Sunnyvale, CA, USA) can be used to deliver a single large intraoperative dose of radiation. As soon as the balloon is inflated, tissue conformance to the surface of the balloon must be checked. Air pockets or fluid/blood collections are deleterious because they push tissue, targeted for treatment, away from the dose cloud, and are to be avoided. The skin thickness in front of the balloon must be evaluated. If the dose is calculated 10 mm from the balloon surface and skin separation is thinner than 10 mm (which is usually the case), then the skin will receive a higher-than-dose prescription. High skin dose will increase the risk of cosmetic failure, telangiectasia, and poor wound healing. There are many publications describing the experience and use of MammoSite (Hologic, Bedford, MA, USA) or Contura (SenoRx, Irvine, CA, USA) as a 10-fraction/5-day PBI.[15] There are no data using these balloon catheters to deliver a single large fraction intraoperatively as part of oncoplastic surgery. Again, the limitations are the lack of a final pathology report to document that the patient is a candidate for PBI, quality assurance, and potential healing problems after a single large fraction of RT with a significant skin dose.

## 12.5 Conclusions

PBI is feasible after oncoplastic surgery. Single-entry balloon and strut-based catheters are not usable after the cavity is closed, but may be feasible as a single intraoperative dose. The data from the randomized intraoperative electron beam Italian trial should shed light on the local control rates, toxicity, and cosmetic outcomes associated with a large single dose of radiation at the time of surgery.

To maximize the possibility of 5-day PBI, we recommend placement of surgical clips of the cavity wall before oncoplastic closure of the cavity, followed by 5-day interstitial brachytherapy.[16] A major advantage of this approach is ensuring the patient is an appropriate candidate for PBI before the treatment is delivered. After reviewing the pathology report, the patient can be scheduled for interstitial brachytherapy 2–6 weeks after oncoplastic surgery. Three-dimensional conformal external beam PBI is also feasible, but the skin dose will be higher than brachytherapy, and the field may be quite large in order to cover 2.5 cm beyond the clips.

As oncoplastic surgery becomes more prevalent, prospective clinical trials will demonstrate the efficacy, toxicity, and cosmetic outcomes of PBI during or after oncoplastic surgery.

## References

1. Boyd NF, Guo H, Martin LJ, *et al.* (2007) Mammographic density and the risk and detection of breast cancer. *N Engl J Med* 356(3):227–236.
2. King TA, Bolton JS, Kuske RR, *et al.* (2000) Long-term results of wide-field brachytherapy as the sole method of radiation therapy after segmental mastectomy for T(is,1,2) breast cancer. *Am J Surg* 180(4):299–304.
3. Vicini FA, Baglan KL, Kestin LL, *et al.* (2001) Accelerated treatment of breast cancer. *J Clin Oncol* 19(7):1993–2001.
4. Arthur DW, Winter K, Kuske RR, *et al.* (2008) A phase II trial of brachytherapy alone after lumpectomy for select breast cancer: Tumor control and survival outcomes of RTOG 95-17. *Int J Radiat Oncol Biol Phys* 72(2): 467–473.
5. Kuske RR, Winter K, Arthur DW, *et al.* (2006) Phase II trial of brachytherapy alone after lumpectomy for select breast cancer: Toxicity analysis of RTOG 95-17. *Int J Radiat Oncol Biol Phys* 65(1):45–51.
6. Beal K, McCormick B, Zelefsky MJ, *et al.* (2007) Single-fraction intraoperative radiotherapy for breast cancer: Early cosmetic results. *Int J Radiat Oncol Biol Phys* 69(1):19–24.
7. Lebovic GS. (2010) Oncoplastic surgery: A creative approach to breast cancer management. *Surg Oncol Clin N Am* 19(3):567–580.

8. Clough KB, Kaufman GJ, Nos C, *et al.* (2010) Improving breast cancer surgery: A classification and quadrant per quadrant atlas for oncoplastic surgery. *Ann Surg Oncol* 17(5):1375–1391.
9. Silverstein MH, Recht A. (2001) Image-detected breast cancer: State of the art diagnosis and treatment. International Breast Cancer Consensus Conference. *J Am Coll Surg* 193(3):297–302.
10. Silverstein MJ, Recht A, Lagios MD, *et al.* (20090 Special report: Consensus Conference III. Image-detected breast cancer: State-of-the-art diagnosis and treatment. *J Am Coll Surg* 209(4):504–520.
11. Kuske RR, Boyer C, Bolton JS. (2004) Long-term results of the Ochsner Clinic prospective phase II breast brachytherapy trial. San Antonio Breast Conference.
12. Chen PY. (2010) A matched pair analysis of partial breast irradiation versus whole breast irradiation at the William Beaumont Hospital, American Brachytherapy Society Annual Meeting.
13. Polgar C, Sulyok Z, Fodor J, *et al.* (2002) Sole brachytherapy of the tumor bed after conservative surgery for T1 breast cancer: Five-year results of a phase I–II study and initial findings of a randomized phase III trial. *J Surg Oncol* 80(3):121–128; discussion 129.
14. Vicini FA, Remouchamps V, Wallace M, *et al.* (2003) Ongoing clinical experience utilizing 3D conformal external beam radiotherapy to deliver partial-breast irradiation in patients with early-stage breast cancer treated with breast-conserving therapy. *Int J Radiat Oncol Biol Phys* 57(5):1247–1253.
15. Nelson JC, Beitsch PD, Vicini FA, *et al.* (2009) Four-year clinical update from the American Society of Breast Surgeons MammoSite brachytherapy trial. *Am J Surg* 198(1):83–91.
16. Kuske RR. (2008, 2009, and 2010) Breast brachytherapy in women with breast cancer treated by oncoplastic breast-conserving techniques. American Society of Breast Disease annual course in Oncoplastic Surgery, Dallas, Texas.

# INDEX